*Free with*

**BD Chaurasia's**

## Human Anatomy | Volumes 3 and 4

**Tenth Edition**

# Workbook of Human Anatomy

Learn | Assess | Practice Activity

As per the latest NMC Guidelines | Competency Based Medical Education (CBME) Curriculum under Graduate Medical Education Regulation

## Head and Neck

## Brain–Neuroanatomy

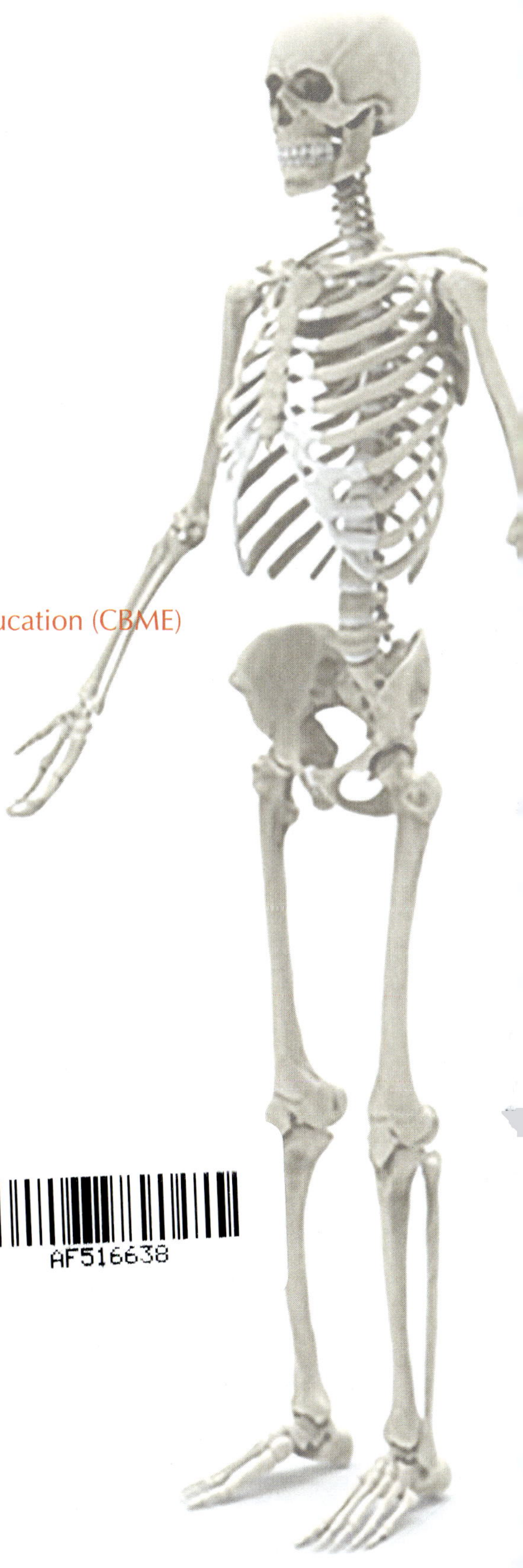

*Free with*

**BD Chaurasia's**

**Human Anatomy** | Volumes 3 and 4

**Tenth Edition**

# Workbook of Human Anatomy

Learn | Assess | Practice Activity

As per the latest NMC Guidelines | Competency Based Medical Education (CBME) Curriculum under Graduate Medical Education Regulation

## Head and Neck

## Brain–Neuroanatomy

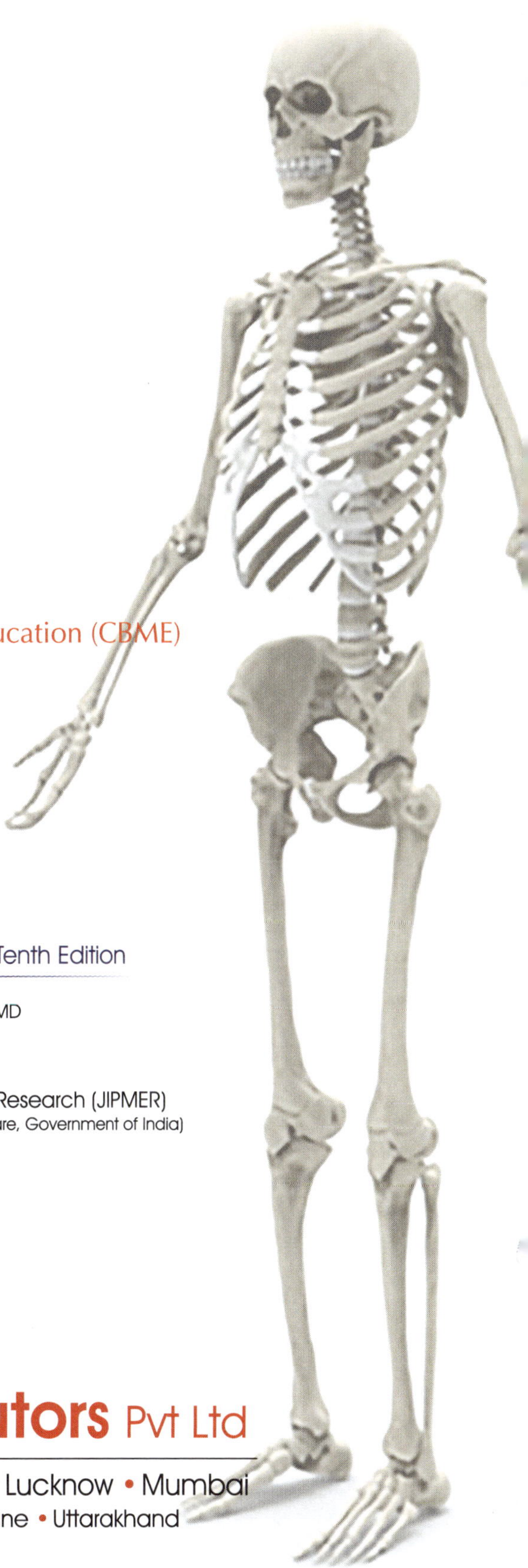


Executive Editor, BD Chaurasia's *Human Anatomy*, Tenth Edition

**Yogesh Ashok Sontakke** MBBS MD

Additional Professor

Department of Anatomy

Jawaharlal Institute of Postgraduate Medical Education and Research (JIPMER)

(An Institute of National Importance under the Ministry of Health and Family Welfare, Government of India)

Puducherry, India



CBSPD

**CBS Publishers & Distributors** Pvt Ltd

New Delhi • Bengaluru • Chennai • Kochi • Kolkata • Lucknow • Mumbai

Gujarat • Hyderabad • Jharkhand • Nagpur • Patna • Pune • Uttarakhand

*Disclaimer*

Science and technology are constantly changing fields. New research and experience broaden the scope of information and knowledge. The author has tried his best in giving information available to him while preparing the material for this book. Although all efforts have been made to ensure optimum accuracy of the material, yet it is quite possible some errors might have been left uncorrected. The publisher, the printer and the author will not be held responsible for any inadvertent errors, omissions or inaccuracies.

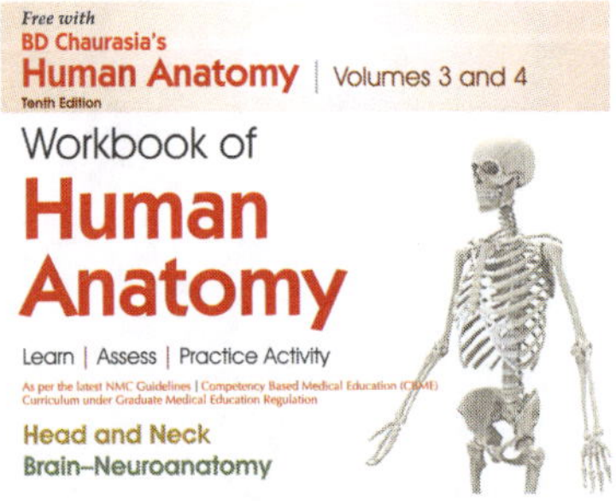


To accompany BD Chaurasia's Human Anatomy Vol 3 and 4

**ISBN:** 978-93-5466-943-9



Published by Satish Kumar Jain and produced by Varun Jain for

**CBS Publishers & Distributors** Pvt Ltd
4819/XI Prahlad Street, 24 Ansari Road, Daryaganj, New Delhi 110 002, India
Ph: 011-23289259, 23266838 Website: www.cbspd.com
e-mail: delhi@cbspd.com

*Corporate Office*: 204 FIE, Industrial Area, Patparganj, Delhi 110 092, India
Ph: 011-4934 4934 Fax: 011-4934 4935 e-mail: publishing@cbspd.com; publicity@cbspd.com

***Branches***

- **Bengaluru:** Seema House 2975, 17th Cross, K.R. Road, Banasankari 2nd Stage, Bengaluru 560 070, Karnataka, India
  Ph: +91-80-26771678/79 Fax: +91-80-26771680 e-mail: bangalore@cbspd.com
- **Chennai:** 18/8B, Subbarayan Street, Shenoy Nagar, Chennai 600 030, Tamil Nadu, India
  Ph: +91-44-42032115, 26681266 e-mail: chennai@cbspd.com
- **Kochi:** 42/1325, 1326, Power House Road, Opposite KSEB, Power House, Ernakulum 682 018, Kochi, Kerala, India
  Ph: +91-484-4059061–65, 67 Fax: +91-484-4059065 e-mail: kochi@cbspd.com
- **Kolkata:** 147, Hind Ceramics Compound, 1st Floor, Nilgunj Road, Belghoria, Kolkata 700 056, West Bengal, India
  Ph: +91-33-25633055/56 e-mail: kolkata@cbspd.com
- **Lucknow:** Basement, Khushnuma Complex, 7 Meerabai Marg (behind Jawahar Bhawan), Lucknow 226 001, UP, India
  Ph: +91-522-4000032 e-mail: tiwari.lucknow@cbspd.com
- **Mumbai:** PWD Shed, Gala No. 25/26, Ramchandra Bhatt Marg, Next JJ Hospital Gate No. 2, Opp. Union Bank of India, Noorbaug, Mumbai 400 009, Maharashtra, India
  Ph: +91-22-66661880/89 e-mail: mumbai@cbspd.com

***Representatives***

- **Gujarat** 0-9879558667
- **Hyderabad** 0-9885175004
- **Jharkhand** 0-9811541605
- **Nagpur** 0-8692091830
- **Patna** 0-9334159340
- **Pune** 0-9664372571
- **Uttarakhand** 0-9716462459

*Printed at*: Thomson Press (India) Ltd., Faridabad, Haryana, India

# Preface

The *Workbook of Human Anatomy* is prepared after discussions with the students to fulfil the requirements of students for examination preparations. This workbook will help the students to achieve the required levels of the given competencies: Knows (K), knows how (KH) and shows how (SH), with the help of included domains of learning, knowledge (K) and skills (S). To fulfil the need for curriculum, requirements of the students and the field of medicine, it is essential for every learner to convert subject knowledge into presentable format in the examinations.

Students face the problem in revision and focusing on the practice of figures and revising the subject. Each book on the anatomy contains thousands of images. It is very difficult to select the figures to be practised. To solve these students' concerns, this *Workbook* has been prepared to help the students by making them aware about practising selected figures for preparation of theory examinations. The students should keep in mind that while answering the questions in the examination about anatomy, if they support the answer by a selected figure, the explanation will be easy and presentable.

To address these issues of the students, this workbook is facilitated with the following features:

1. Clinicoanatomical problems will help to sensitize the students to Early Clinical Exposure.
2. MCQs will help in analysing the understanding of the subject.
3. Question Bank will help to prepare for upcoming academic examinations.
4. Spotters will help to prepare for practical examinations.
5. Answer Keys will help to cross-check and self-assessments.

Always read a complete textbook for getting better knowledge and generating perfect concepts of the subject. ***Cadavers and dissections are the best teachers of human anatomy***. Due to increasing number of students in the medical colleges and less availability of cadavers, under the expertise of teachers, the students can utilize their spare time in the dissection hall to complete this workbook. It will help in consolidation of the knowledge and better understanding of the structures. Due to space constrain, all practice figures are not included in this Workbook. Students are advised to practice additional images in their practice notebooks.

For any suggestions, please write at dryogeshas@gmail.com

**Yogesh Ashok Sontakke**

# Instructions to Students

1. Read the theory part from the main textbook before starting to solve the workbook.
2. *Clinicoanatomical problems*: Read these problems carefully. Write precise answers. Use separate sheet of copy for writing in details.
3. *Practice figures*: As we are aware that many students are good in drawings and to avoid difficulty of initial stages of drawings, the workbook is provided with dotted outlines of practice figures. Trace these lines with suitable colour pencils and shade the figures. Refer the main Textbook before colouring the figures. Label the figures with good handwriting.
4. *MCQs*: Tick the single best correct option in the workbook. Some diagram based MCQs are introduced to align with CBME pattern.
5. *Question bank*: It will give orientation towards upcoming academic examinations. Use separate copy to solve the following questions. Maintain this copy properly so that it can be referred during subject revision.
6. *Spotters*: These will give orientation towards practical examinations. Solve them on a separate sheet.
7. *Answer keys*: Match your answers with the provided key. Self-evaluation is the best method for progress.
8. *eSmartQuiz – Online MCQ test*: Scan the QR code for online MCQ test. Fill the required details and solve the test.

   Always keep in mind "*Practice is essential and integral part of academics. Hard work is the path for success*".

**Yogesh Ashok Sontakke**

# Contents

# *eSmartQuiz* – Online MCQ Test

After attending the class, students should go through the "*eSmartQuiz* – Online MCQ test" for the following reasons:

- *Reinforcement of Learning*: The "*eSmartQuiz* – Online MCQ test" provides an opportunity to reinforce learning after attending a class or reading a book. It helps to assess understanding and retention of concepts, to solidify knowledge and identify areas that need further revision or clarification.
- *Assessment of Comprehension*: The "*eSmartQuiz* – Online MCQ test" is an effective tool to assess comprehension of the subject matter and to demonstrate the ability to apply the concepts learned in the class.
- *Enhancement of Attention and Critical Thinking*: The "*eSmartQuiz* – Online MCQ test" will help to make students attentive for the class and to enhance critical thinking skills by selecting the most appropriate answer among the given options.

Each *eSmartQuiz* test consists of 10 MCQ, mostly image-based, and the students can see their scores at the end of each test. These questions will be modified after a certain interval. Use the given links or scan the QR code (given in each chapter) for the test. One student can solve each test only one time.

| *Chapter* | *Link for **eSmartQuiz*** |
|---|---|
| **Head and Neck** | |
| 1. Osteology of Head and Neck | https://forms.gle/L23dCS6nuUdcH4416 |
| 2. Scalp, Temple and Face | https://forms.gle/JCQ9kMV1n5q3hwHd6 |
| 3. Side of the Neck | https://forms.gle/o7xkkfE8nZwp7qUC6 |
| 4. Anterior Region of the Neck | https://forms.gle/VzXQVfSfbTaHJZTn7 |
| 5. Parotid Region | https://forms.gle/uKsU6corLTTnBovz5 |
| 6. Temporal and Infratemporal Regions | https://forms.gle/iP5JkDtKtrRL8r1r8 |
| 7. Submandibular Region | https://forms.gle/3NVu6uePp3ZgbUv57 |
| 8. Structures in the Neck | https://forms.gle/rukg8W5wummqvsnv9 |
| 9. Prevertebral and Paravertebral Regions | https://forms.gle/gVEpDdaTY7kvFWJ99 |
| 10. Back of the Neck | https://forms.gle/nPGqbURZPH2i7hg77 |
| 11. Contents of Vertebral Canal | https://forms.gle/vxZuN9BhChfqYHa36 |
| 12. Cranial Cavity | https://forms.gle/bwgzsWSvQ9HV6KSz9 |
| 13. Contents of the Orbit | https://forms.gle/1KgWiySrEVWFhRCUA |
| 14. Mouth and Pharynx | https://forms.gle/F74Vwpj43aHSBxr86 |
| 15. Nose, Paranasal Sinuses and Pterygopalatine Fossa | https://forms.gle/tMAGush9LAF929FF8 |
| 16. Larynx | https://forms.gle/VyjBKNLUNb4FzEvdA |
| 17. Tongue | https://forms.gle/cT17eXaE9fo1HYKNA |
| 18. Ear | https://forms.gle/618J9JzvQC4Sm9229 |
| 19. Eyeball | https://forms.gle/iVm65VU6LSHKhRsu5 |
| 20. Surface Marking and Radiological Anatomy | https://forms.gle/MEpq8w8CXdjvgRyS8 |

(Contd.)

(*Contd.*)

| *Chapter* | *Link for* **eSmartQuiz** |
|---|---|
| **Brain–Neuroanatomy** | |
| 1. Organisation of Nervous System | https://forms.gle/q3QXQaymKrN8LpvB8 |
| 2. Peripheral Nerves and Ganglia | https://forms.gle/ZdAcAbiBLx22dcP19 |
| 3. Receptors | https://forms.gle/1By6ddQt6Y1Vf7saA |
| 4. Meninges of the Brain and Cerebrospinal Fluid | https://forms.gle/KsXnZzsHqy6ghy5XA |
| 5. Spinal Cord | https://forms.gle/M5b5xRmq52m64H24A |
| 6. Cranial Nerves | https://forms.gle/H1ws2DKLCctwm8Gx7 |
| 7. Brainstem | https://forms.gle/J5E9oiZZ4sZpZzJV6 |
| 8. Cerebellum | https://forms.gle/X1b5HvoSK3TqDHSm6 |
| 9. Fourth Ventricle | https://forms.gle/FWf7GEgYhPxzUNSS6 |
| 10. Diencephalon and Third Ventricle | https://forms.gle/pAsf7NtBmtYSE51r6 |
| 11. Cerebrum, Basal Nuclei and White Matter | https://forms.gle/tYvNGezPahWx5dV56 |
| 12. Lateral Ventricle and Limbic System | https://forms.gle/JdLkLaob4K1eMdzy8 |
| 13. Some Neural Pathways and Reticular Formation | https://forms.gle/E4fzgQp2NKfNkb3W9 |
| 14. Blood Supply of Brain | https://forms.gle/8pbcViRGCJ1N67kK6 |
| 15. Surface Marking and Radiological Anatomy of Nervous System | https://forms.gle/K5rzTmY6hD8pM6nn9 |
| 16. Autonomic Nervous System | https://forms.gle/3q9bCZtNHiA27UDU6 |
| 17. Development of Nervous System | https://forms.gle/UMXxbzcC1hA1Rpg88 |

# Head and Neck

Chapter 1

# Osteology of Head and Neck

eSmartQuiz

## CLINICOANATOMICAL PROBLEMS

### Clinical Case 1

A 25-year-old male was hit on the temple during a cricket, resulting in an injury at the pterion. He briefly lost consciousness but felt fine afterwards. Later, he developed a severe headache and confusion. At the hospital, a CT scan revealed an **extradural haematoma**. Immediate surgical intervention was required to evacuate the haematoma and stop the arterial bleeding.

1. What is pterion?
2. Which vessels most probably got damaged in this case?

*Explanation*

1. ______________________________

2. ______________________________

### Clinical Case 2

A 2-week-old newborn presented with fever and irritability. Suspecting meningitis, the paediatrician collected the cerebrospinal fluid (CSF) sample through the anterior **fontanelle**. The results confirmed the diagnosis, allowing for prompt initiation of appropriate antibiotic therapy.

1. What is anterior fontanelle?
2. When it closes?
3. Name other fontanelle of the skull.

*Explanation*

1. ______________________________

2. ______________________________

3. ______________________________

## PRACTICE FIGURES

(Label the practice figures)

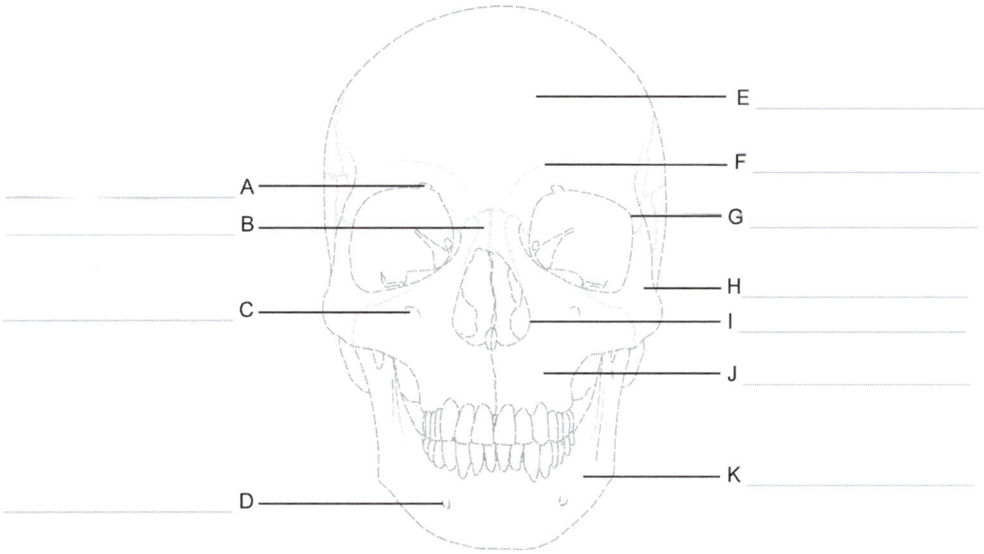


**Practice Fig. 1.1:** Norma frontalis

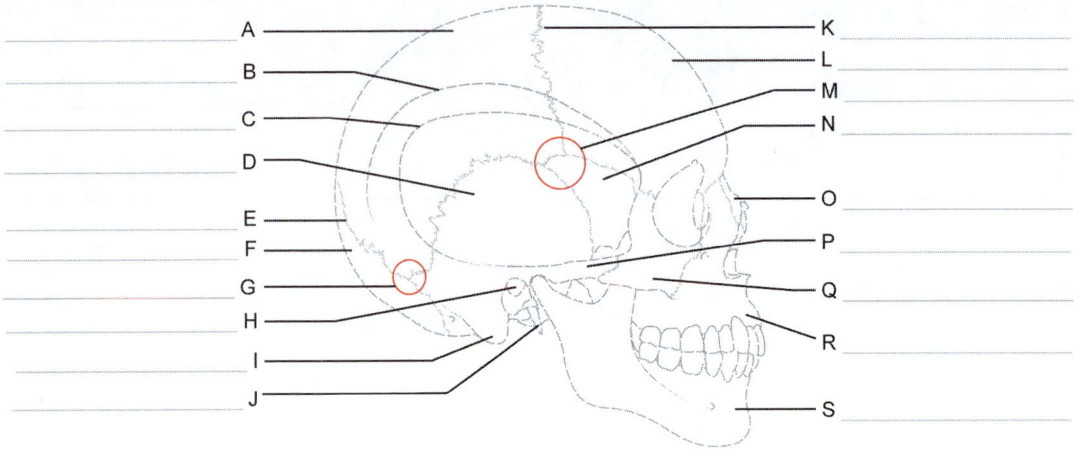


**Practice Figure 1.2:** Norma lateralis

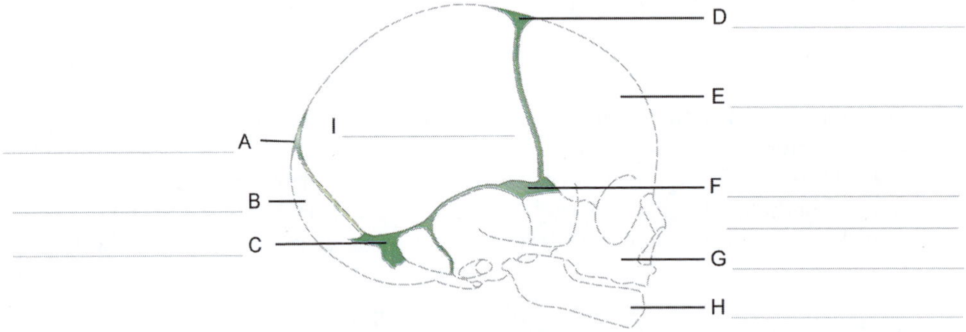


**Practice Figure 1.3:** Fontanelles of skull

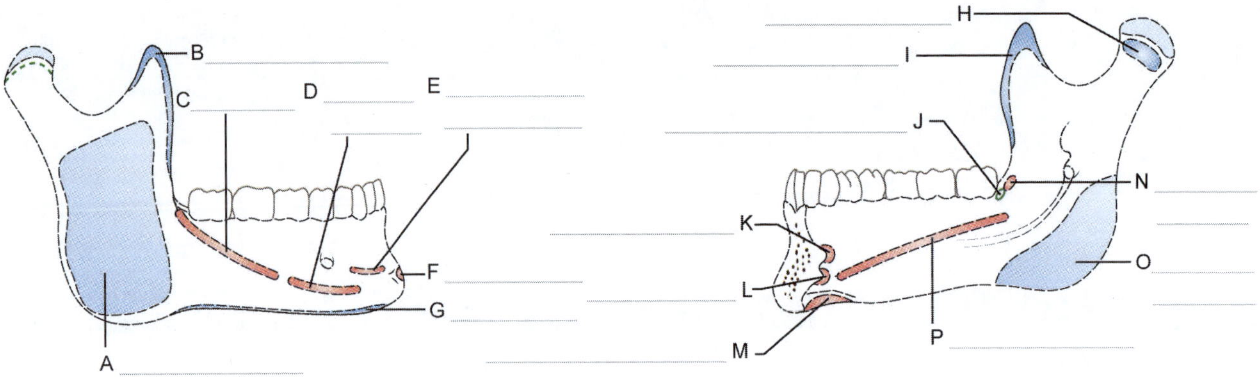


**Practice Figure 1.4:** Attachments of the mandible

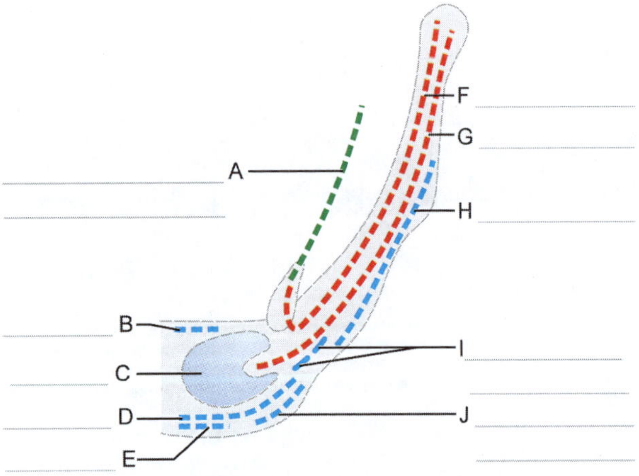


**Practice Figure 1.5:** Attachments of the hyoid bone

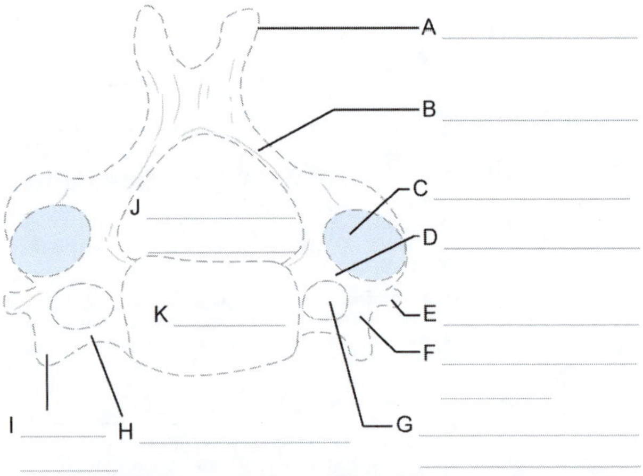


**Practice Figure 1.6:** Typical cervical vertebra

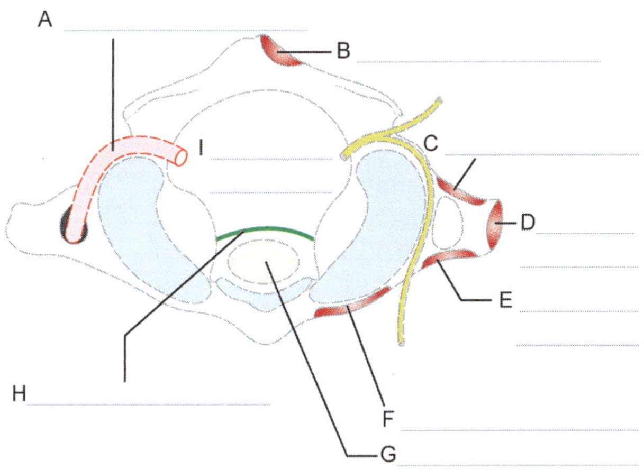


**Practice Figure 1.7:** Relations of atlas vertebra

## MULTIPLE CHOICE QUESTIONS

(Tick the single best correct option)

1. Identify X in the below image.

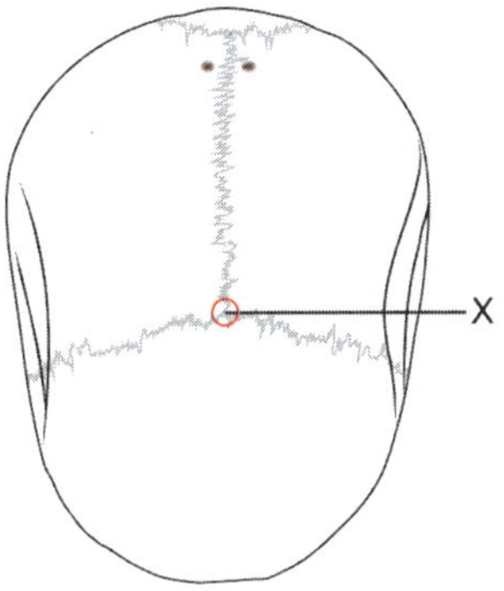


   a. Bregma b. Obelion
   c. Lambda d. Pterion

2. All of the following structures form the boundaries of McEwan's triangle, EXCEPT:
   a. Supramastoid crest
   b. Posterosuperior margin of the external meatus
   c. Lateral wall of the tympanic cavity
   d. Suprameatal spine

3. The mastoid foramen transmits ___________.
   a. Facial nerve
   b. Auricular branch of the vagus nerve
   c. Greater auricular nerve
   d. Mastoid emissary vein

4. Identify the clinical condition shown in the following image.

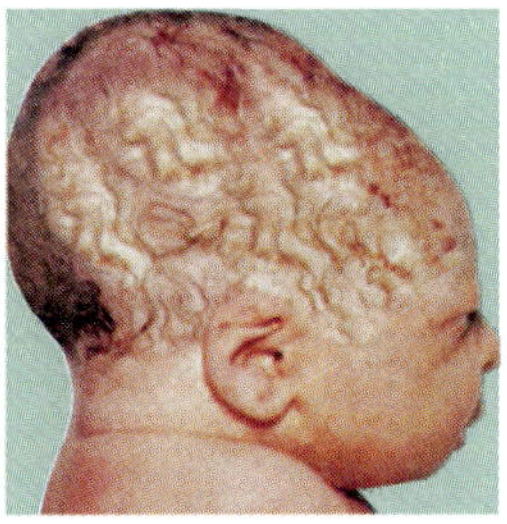

   a. Posterior fossa tumour b. Caput cephalohematoma
   c. Caput succedaneum d. Caput medusae

5. A 3-week-old newborn was brought to the emergency department by her parents. Child was fussy, vomiting after every feed. On examination-anterior fontanelle is bulged. What could be the cause?
   a. Arteriovenous malformation
   b. Raised intracranial pressure
   c. Cerebral haemorrhage
   d. Severe dehydration

6. Which of the following structures is damaged in the fracture occurring at the X-marked site?

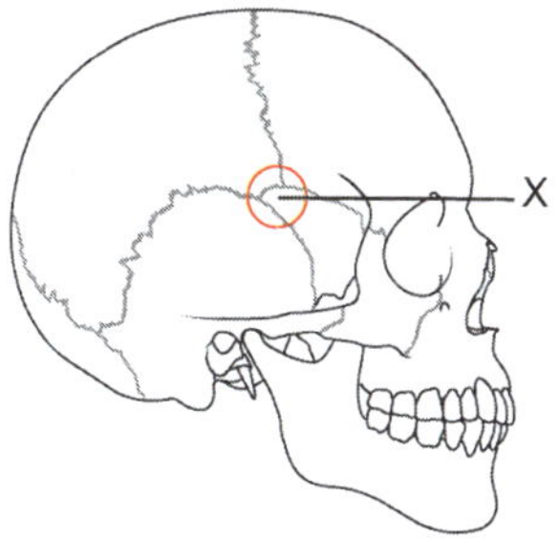


   a. Facial nerve
   b. Olfactory bulb
   c. Middle meningeal artery
   d. Basilar artery

7. All of the following structures are content of the foramen ovale, EXCEPT?
   a. Maxillary nerve
   b. Accessory meningeal artery
   c. Lesser petrosal nerve
   d. Emissary vein

8. Name the structure marked as X.

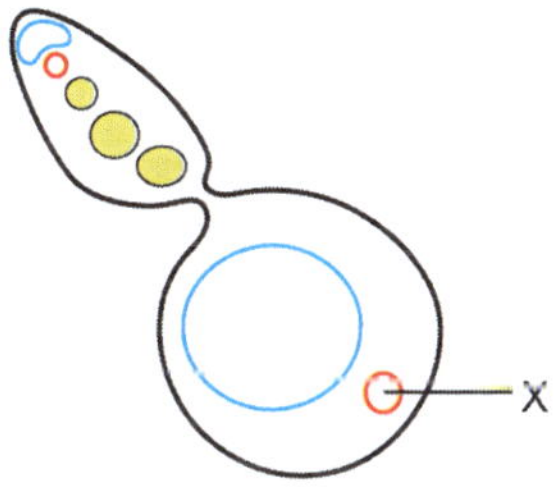


   a. Meningeal branch of pharyngeal artery
   b. Meningeal branch of occipital artery
   c. Anterior meningeal artery
   d. Posterior meningeal artery

9. Which of the following muscle gets inserted at the X-marked site of the outer surface of the mandible?

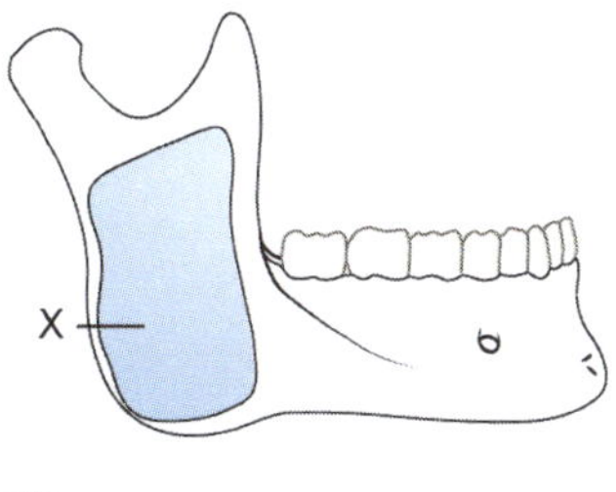


   a. Buccinator
   b. Masseter
   c. Orbicularis oris
   d. Medial pterygoid muscle

10. Which nerve passes through the marked foramen?

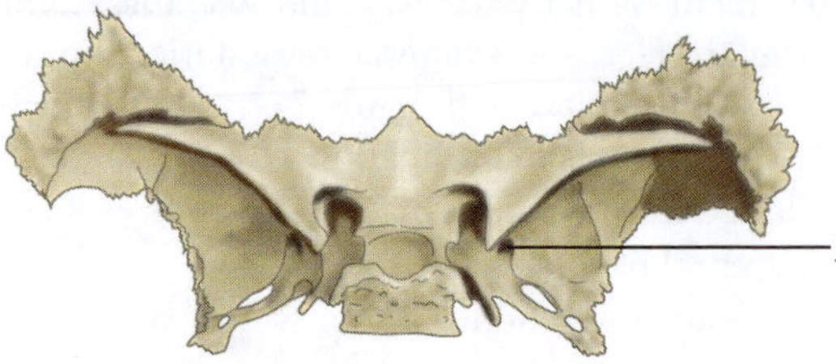


a. Facial nerve
b. Mandibular nerve
c. Abducens nerve
d. Maxillary nerve

11. All of the following are features of atlas bone, EXCEPT:
a. It is ring-shaped and has neither a body nor a spine
b. Its anterior surface bears an oval facet that articulates with the dens
c. The medial surface of the lateral mass is marked by a small roughened tubercle
d. The transverse process projects laterally from the lateral mass

12. Cervical rib commonly arises from ___________ vertebra.
a. C4
b. C3
c. C7
d. C5

13. Scaphocephaly or boat-shaped skull is due to premature synostosis in ___________ suture.
a. Coronal
b. Sagittal
c. Lambdoid
d. Temporal

## QUESTION BANK

(Use separate copy to solve the following questions)

Q 1. Mention the structures passing through the following foramina:
a. Foramen magnum
b. Jugular foramen
c. Superior orbital fissure
d. Foramen ovale
e. Internal acoustic meatus

Q 2. Mention the attachments of:
a. Spine of sphenoid
b. Styloid process
c. Mastoid process

Q 3. Draw a well-labelled diagram showing parts and attachments of the hyoid bone.

Q 4. Write a short notes on:
a. Fontanelle of skull
b. Age changes in mandible
c. Identifying features of the 1st, 2nd, and typical cervical vertebrae

Chapter

2

# Scalp, Temple and Face

eSmartQuiz

## CLINICOANATOMICAL PROBLEMS

### Clinical Case 1

A 32-year-old woman suffered a deep laceration behind her right ear in a car accident. She immediately experienced facial drooping and inability to close her eye on the right side. There was overflowing of tears on the right cheek and saliva dribbling from his right angle of the mouth. At the hospital, examination revealed injury to the right facial nerve at its exist through the skull.

1. Name the foramen through which the facial nerve comes out of the skull.
2. Name the muscle which get paralysed and produces: a. inability to close the eyes, b. drooling of saliva from angle of mouth.

#### Explanation

1. 

2. a. 

   b. 

### Clinical Case 2

A 40-year-old man fell from a ladder, hitting his head on the ground. He presented with a deep scalp laceration which bleed profusely, and swelling around his left eye, which turned black and blue.

1. Why the eye turned black in this case?
2. Why the scalp wound bleed profusely?

#### Explanation

1. 

2. 

### Clinical Case 3

A 28-year-old woman developed a painful boil on her upper lip. Despite antibiotic treatment, the infection spread rapidly, causing severe facial swelling and fever. She was admitted to the hospital where she developed severe headache and neck stiffness. A lumbar puncture confirmed meningitis.

1. What is the dangerous area of the face?
2. How the infection from the upper lip spread to the meninges in this case?

#### Explanation

1. 

2. 

### Clinical Case 4

A full-term male newborn required vacuum assistance during delivery. Post-delivery examination revealed a diffuse, fluctuant swelling on his head extending from the orbital ridges anteriorly to the nape of the neck posteriorly. The swelling was well-defined and did not cross suture lines.

1. What is the name for the swelling in this case?
2. What is its anatomical basis?
3. Is it usually present bilaterally?

#### Explanation

1. 

2. 

3. 

## PRACTICE FIGURES

(Label the practice figures)

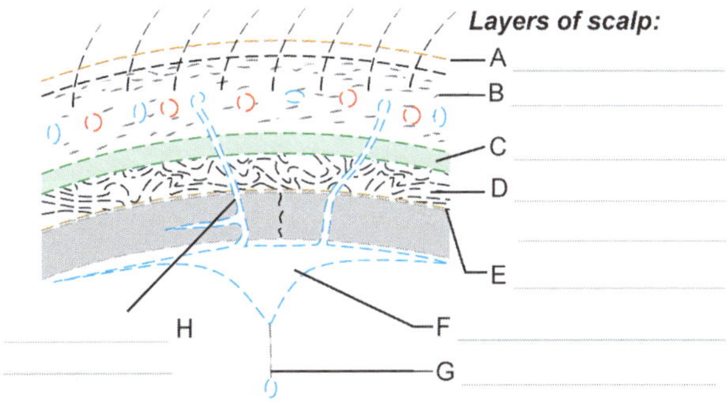


**Practice Figure 2.1:** Layers of scalp

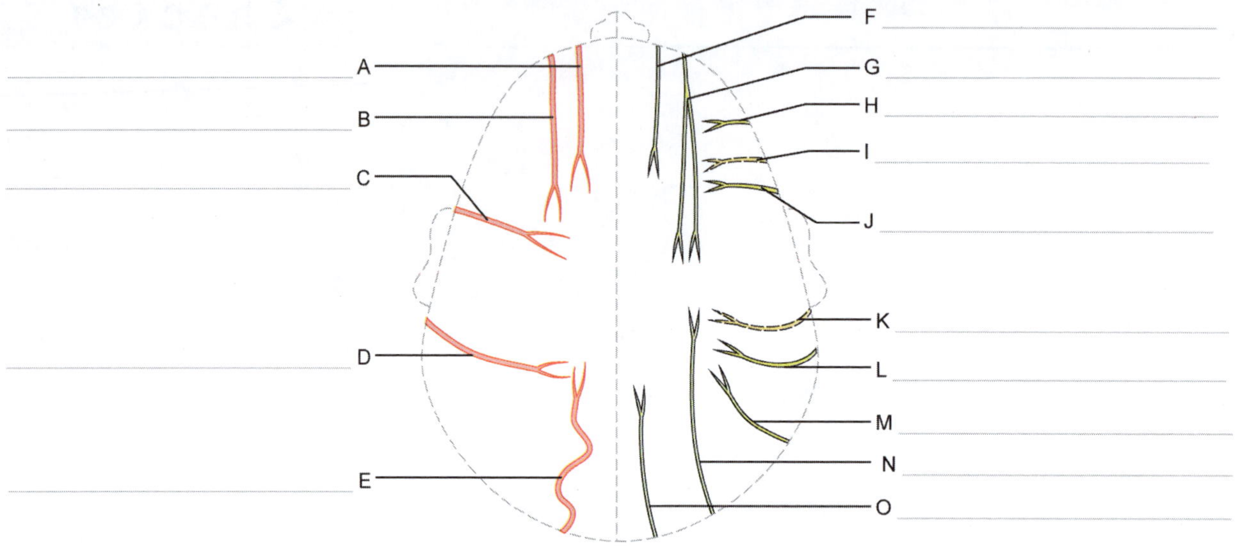


Practice Figure 2.2: Arterial and nerve supply of scalp and superficial temporal region

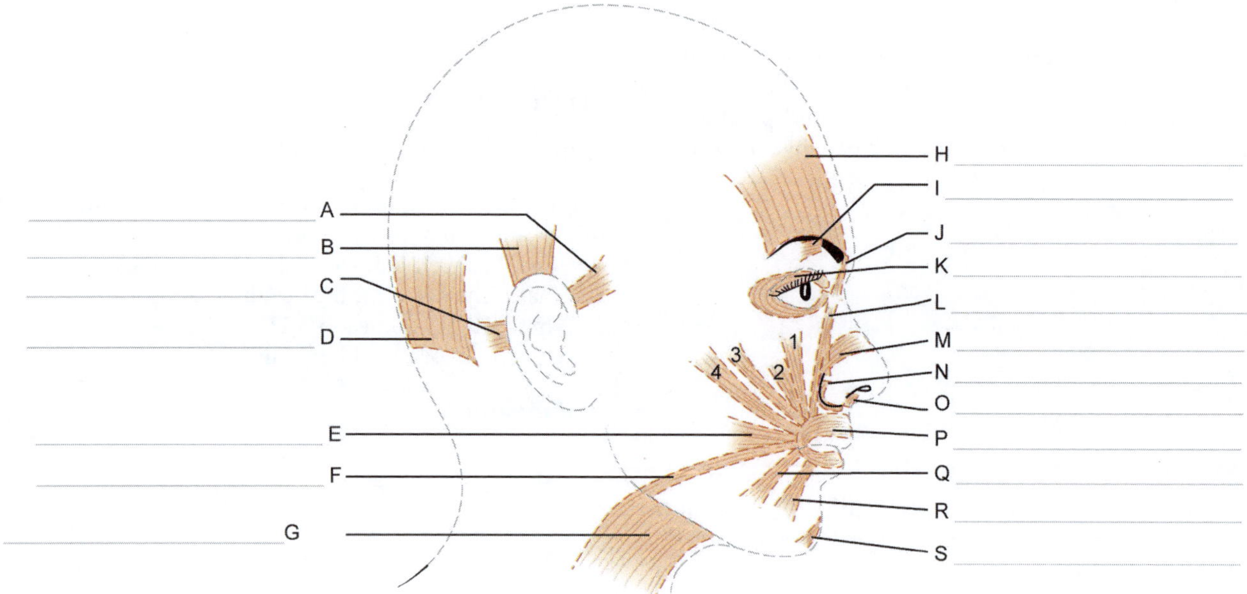


Practice Figure 2.3: Muscles of facial expression (1: levator labii superioris, 2: levator anguli oris, 3: zygomaticus minor, 4: zygomaticus major)

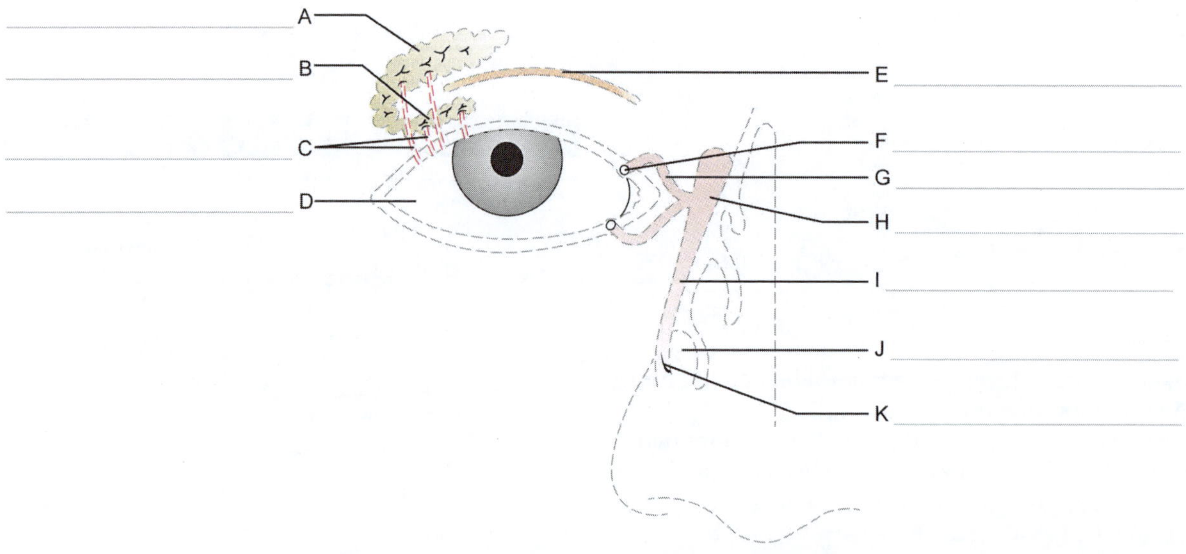


Practice Figure 2.4: Components of lacrimal apparatus

## MULTIPLE CHOICE QUESTIONS

(Tick the single best correct option)

1. Which of the following is known as the dangerous layer of scalp?
   a. Connective tissue  b. Aponeurosis
   c. Loose areolar tissue  d. Pericranium
2. Which of the following is not a modification of deep fascia in face?
   a. Parotid fascia  b. Temporal fascia
   c. Buccopharyngeal fascia  d. Pterygoid fascia
3. Name the structure marked by X in the following picture:

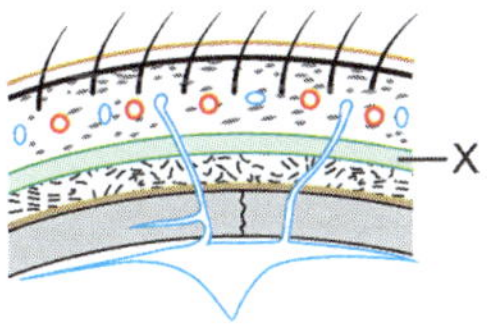


   a. Loose areolar tissue  b. Connective tissue
   c. Superficial fascia  d. Epicranial aponeurosis
4. Which of the following muscles is helpful in whistling?
   a. Orbicularis oris  b. Buccinator
   c. Levator labii superioris  d. Zygomaticus major
5. Which muscle is responsible for the following expression?

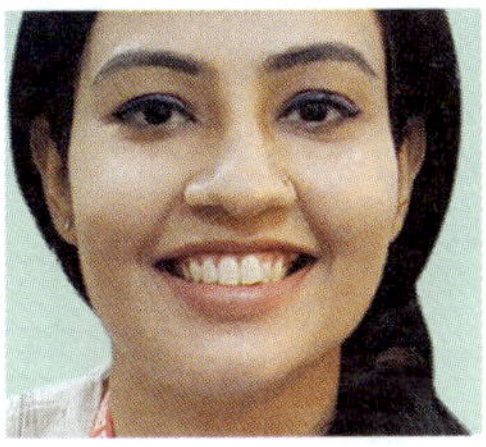

   a. Orbicularis oris  b. Buccinator
   c. Zygomaticus major  d. Lateral pterygoid muscle
6. A 18-year-old boy came to medicine clinic with right side sudden facial weakness and drooling of saliva from his right angle of the mouth. What is the likely nerve affected in this condition?
   a. Facial nerve  b. Mandibular nerve
   c. Maxillary nerve  d. Trigeminal nerve
7. What is the significance of the highlighted area?

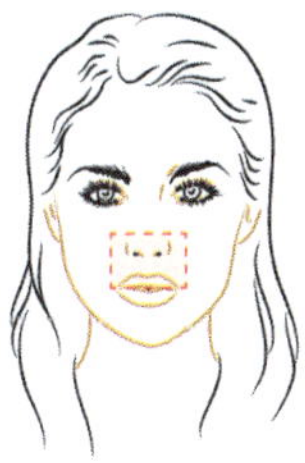

   a. Rich nerve supply
   b. Anastomosis of blood vessels
   c. Communication of facial veins to deep veins
   d. Lymphatic drainage is absent
8. Pick out the incorrect statement about the nasolacrimal duct.
   a. It begins at the lower end of the lacrimal sac, runs downwards, backwards and laterally.
   b. It opens into the middle meatus of the nose.
   c. Valve of Hasner forms the imperfect valve in the lower end of the duct.
   d. It is about 18 mm long.
9. The involuntary part of levator palpebrae superioris is supplied by __________.
   a. Parasympathetic fibre
   b. Lacrimal nerve
   c. Sympathetic fibre
   d. Zygomaticofacial nerve
10. A 57-year-old female came to a neurology clinic with complaints of severe stabbing pain on the left side of her face for the past several months lasting for a few seconds to minutes before subsiding. It is triggered by chewing, talking, or touching her face. What is the likely diagnosis?
    a. Glossopharyngeal neuralgia
    b. Trigeminal neuralgia
    c. Bell's palsy
    d. Migraine
11. __________ pierces the buccinator muscle.
    a. Facial artery
    b. Facial vein
    c. Buccal branch of facial nerve
    d. Marginal mandibular nerve

## QUESTION BANK

(Use separate copy to solve the following questions)

Q 1. Describe the layers of scalp.

Q 2. Write a short notes on:
   a. Blood supply of scalp and its clinical significance.
   b. Lacrimal apparatus
   c. Nerve supply of face
   d. Dangerous area of face
   e. Facial artery
   f. Buccinator muscle
   g. Orbicularis oris muscle

Q 3. Explain the anatomical basis for:
   a. Black eye
   b. Profuse bleeding from scalp wounds
   c. Safety valve haematoma
   d. Caput succedaneum.

Chapter

# 3

# Side of the Neck

eSmartQuiz

## CLINICOANATOMICAL PROBLEM

### Clinical Case 1

A 22-year-old male sustained a sports injury to the posterior triangle of the neck. On examination, there was paralysis of the trapezius muscle with sparing of the sternocleidomastoid muscle function. The clinical findings included shoulder droop and difficulty in raising the affected arm above the shoulder level.

1. Which nerve got damaged in the above-mentioned case?
2. Why there was shoulder droop and difficulty in raising the affected arm?
3. Why only trapezius muscle got paralysed and not the sternocleidomastoid muscle?

### *Explanation*

1. ______________________________

2. ______________________________

3. ______________________________

## PRACTICE FIGURES

(Label the practice figures)

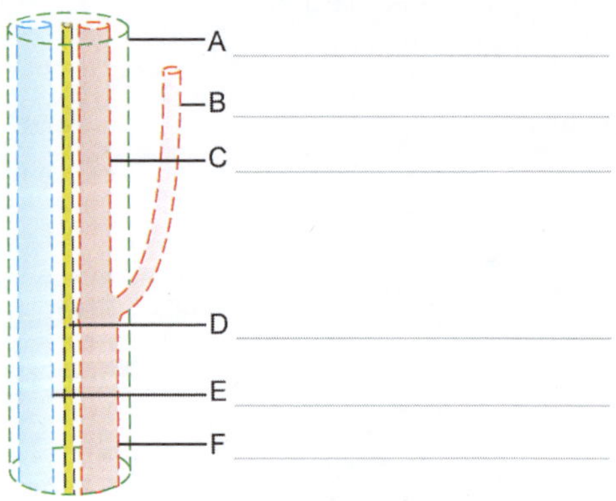


**Practice Figure 3.1:** Carotid sheath

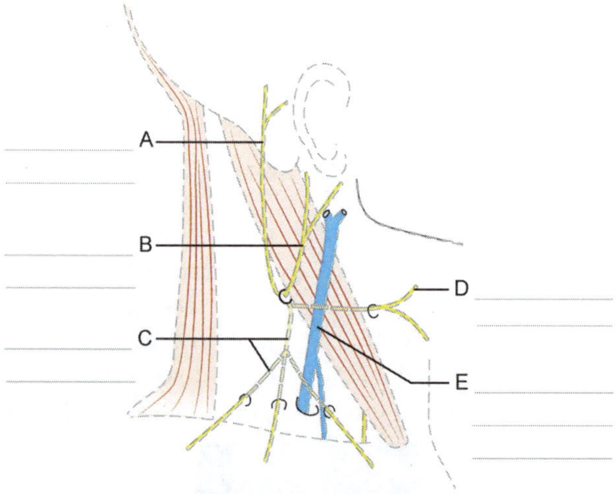


**Practice Figure 3.2:** Roof of the posterior triangle

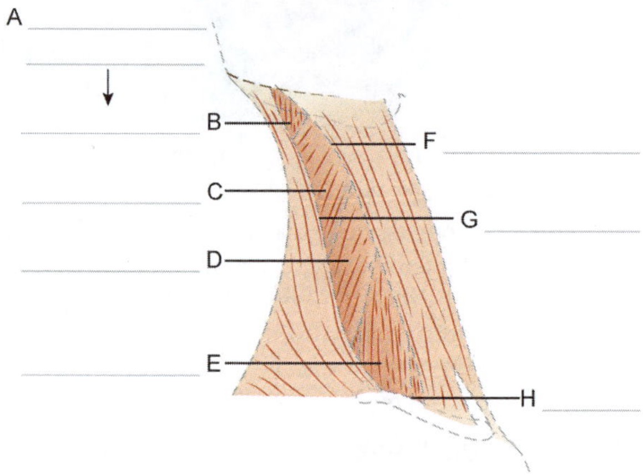


**Practice Figure 3.3:** Floor of the posterior

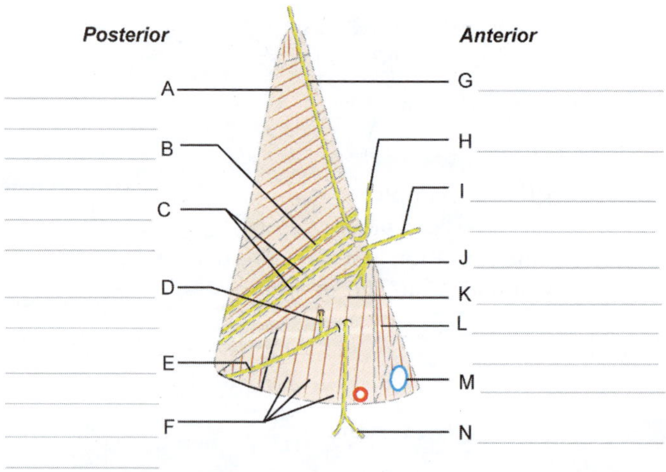


**Practice Figure 3.4:** The contents of posterior triangle of neck

## MULTIPLE CHOICE QUESTIONS

(Tick the single best correct option)

1. Which of the following muscles is the important landmark between the anterior and posterior triangles?
   a. Sternocleidomastoid
   b. Sternohyoid
   c. Trapezius
   d. Superior belly of omohyoid
2. Which among the following is a subcutaneous muscle?
   a. Omohyoid
   b. Sternocleidomastoid
   c. Trapezius
   d. Platysma
3. All of the following are contents of suprasternal space of burns, EXCEPT:
   a. Clavicular heads of the right and left sternocleido-mastoid muscles
   b. Jugular venous arch
   c. Lymph node
   d. Interclavicular ligament
4. Name the structure marked by X in the following picture.

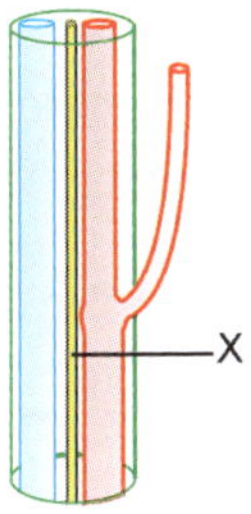


   a. Recurrent laryngeal nerve
   b. Hypoglossal nerve
   c. Vagus nerve
   d. Spinal accessory nerve
5. Identify the structure marked as X in the below image.

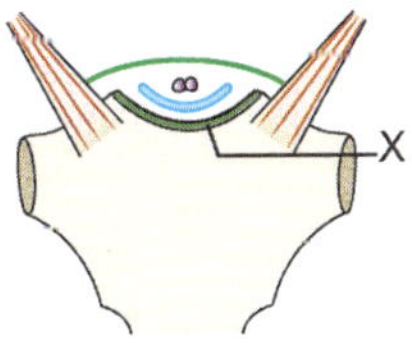


   a. Interclavicular ligament
   b. Investing layer of deep cervical fascia
   c. Anterior longitudinal ligament
   d. Ligament of the dens
6. A 6-week-old male infant was brought to the paediatric clinic by his parents, with complaints of the head position of the baby. On examination, the paediatrician noted that the infant's head is tilted to the right side. The range of motion of the neck is decreased, especially when trying to turn the head to the left. What is the most likely diagnosis?
   a. Congenital myotonic dystrophy
   b. Congenital torticollis
   c. Congenital fibre type disproportion
   d. Becker muscular dystrophy
7. Pick out the incorrect statement about the retropharyngeal space.
   a. It acts as a bursa for expansion of pharynx during deglutition.
   b. The anterior boundary is formed by buccopharyngeal fascia.
   c. The inferior boundary is open and continuous with superior mediastinum.
   d. It is a potential space for tumour to develop.
8. Which anatomical abnormality leads to dysphagia lusoria?
   a. Aortic aneurysm
   b. Aberrant subclavian artery
   c. Oesophageal atresia
   d. Patent ductus arteriosus
9. Dorsal scapular nerve supplies ____________ muscle.
   a. Supraspinatus
   b. Teres major
   c. Rhomboid major
   d. Infraspinatus
10. Spinal root of accessory nerve innervates ____________ muscle.
    a. Serratus anterior
    b. Stylohyoid
    c. Styloglossus
    d. Sternocleidomastoid

## QUESTION BANK

(Use separate copy to solve the following questions)

Q 1. Describe the posterior triangle of neck under the following headings: Boundaries, roof, floor, contents, and applied aspects.

Q 2. Write a short notes on:
   a. Investing layer of deep cervical fascia
   b. Lateral and retropharyngeal space
   c. Carotid sheath
   d. Suprasternal space
   e. Ligament of Berry
   f. Sternocleidomastoid muscle.

Q 3. Write an anatomical basis for:
   a. Wry neck
   b. Painful parotid swelling
   c. Thyroid gland moves with deglutition.

Chapter

# 4

eSmartQuiz

# Anterior Region of the Neck

## CLINICOANATOMICAL PROBLEMS

### Clinical Case 1

A 25-year-old man experienced recurrent episodes of syncope while shaving. During evaluation, he was diagnosed with carotid sinus syndrome. Despite conservative management, his symptoms persisted. Consequently, he underwent periarterial neurectomy of the carotid sinus. Following the procedure, he had no further syncopal episodes and resumed normal activities without complications.

1. What is carotid sinus?
2. In this case, why there were recurrent episodes of syncope while shaving?
3. What is periarterial neurectomy?
4. How will periarterial neurectomy prevent syncope in carotid sinus syndrome?

### Explanation

1. ______________________________

2. ______________________________

3. ______________________________

4. ______________________________

### Clinical Case 2

During abdominal surgery, the anaesthetist monitored the patient's pulse by palpating arteries in the head and neck region while sitting at the head of the table. This ensured the patient's vital signs remained stable throughout the procedure.

1. What was the artery the anaesthetist was palpating and where?
2. Name the other palpable arteries in the head and neck region.
3. Which is the commonly palpated artery in the body during clinical examination?

### Explanation

1. ______________________________

2. ______________________________

3. ______________________________

### Clinical Case 3

A 20-year-old male was brought to the hospital with a severe injury in the lower part of the neck after a knife attack. She was breathless, cyanotic, and hypotensive. The physician identified a vein injury with profuse bleeding and suspected an air embolism.

1. Name the probable veins that was injured in this case.
2. What is air embolism?
3. What is the anatomical reason for the inability of this vein to contract after injury?

### Explanation

1. ______________________________

2. ______________________________

3. ______________________________

## PRACTICE FIGURES

(Label the practice figures)

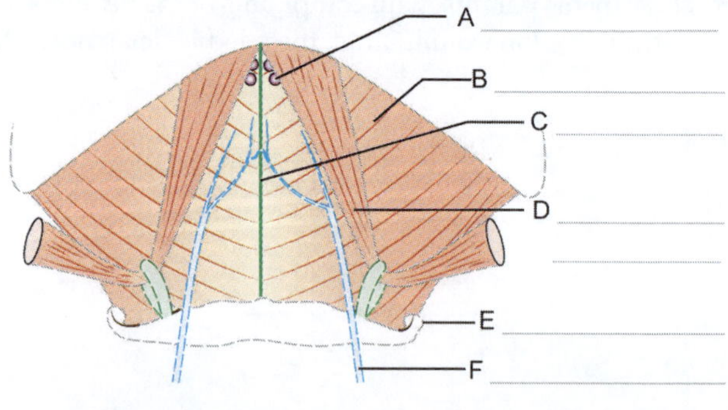


**Practice Figure 4.1:** Boundaries and contents of the submental triangle

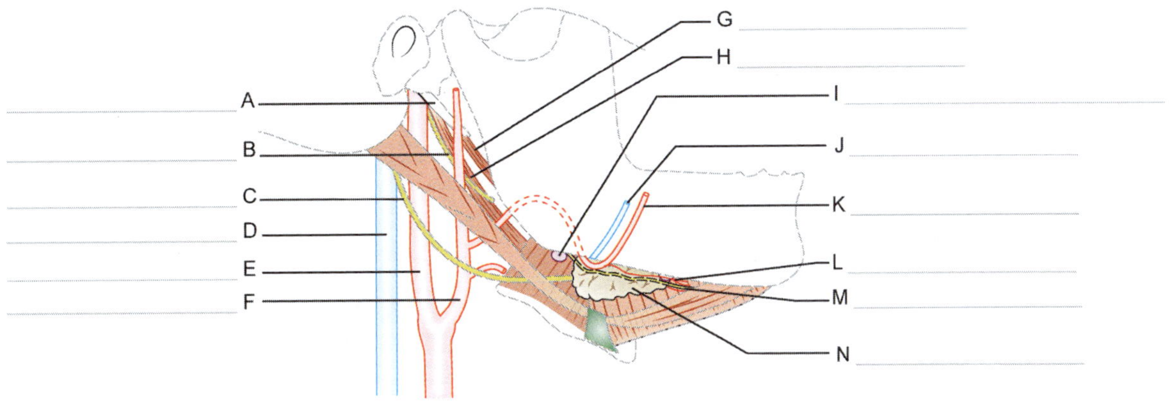


**Practice Figure 4.2:** Contents of the digastric triangle

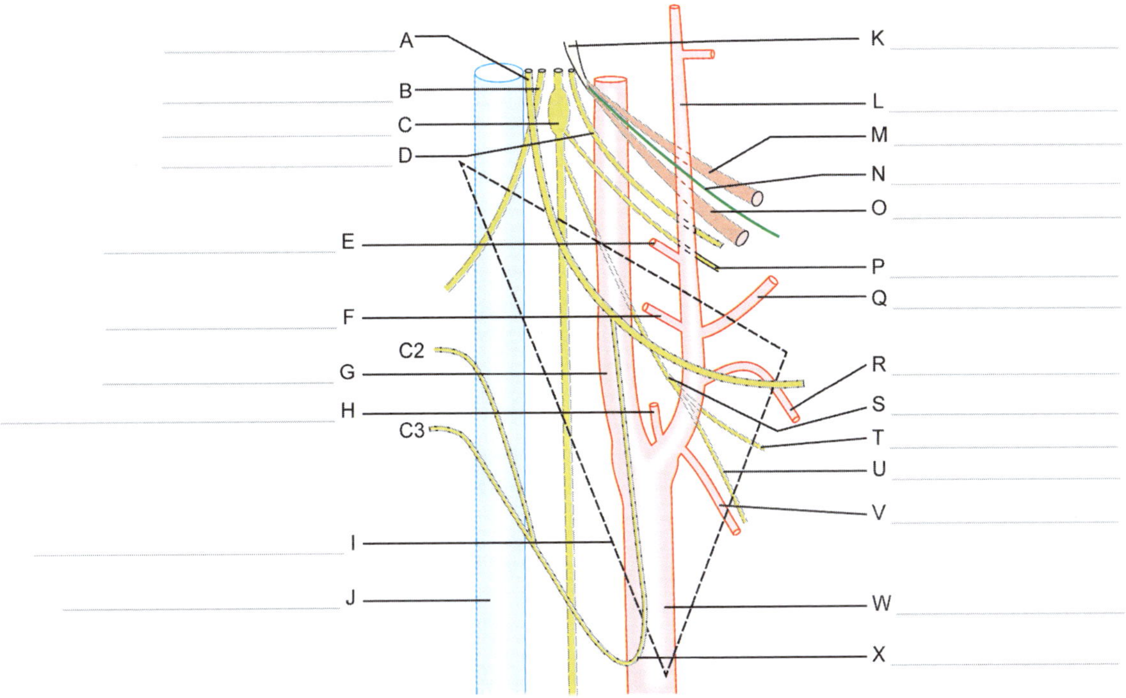


**Practice Figure 4.3:** The IXth, Xth, XIth and XIIth cranial nerves and their branches related to the carotid arteries and to the internal jugular vein

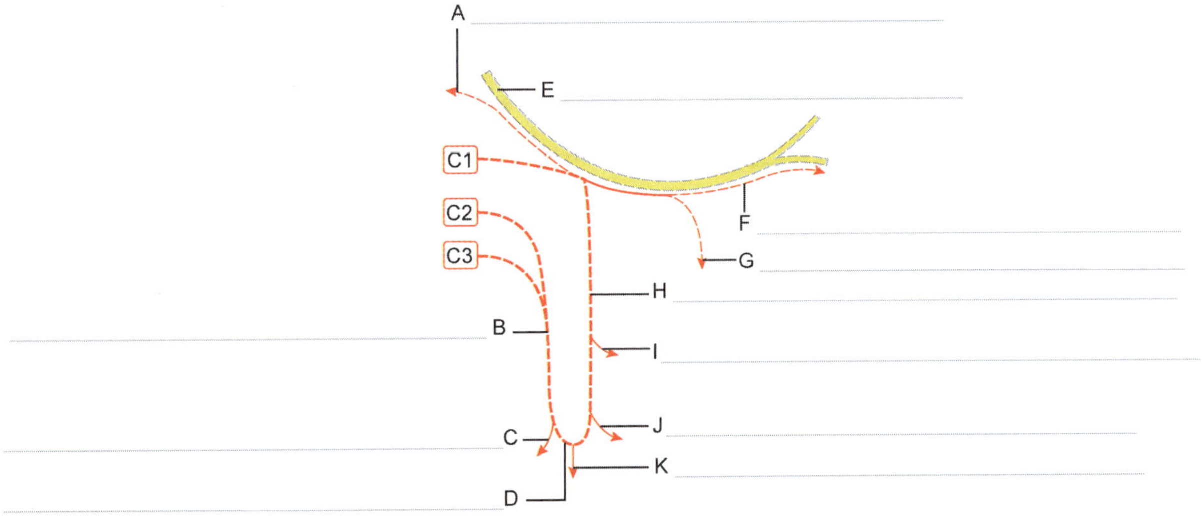


**Practice Figure 4.4:** Ansa cervicalis and branches of the first cervical nerve distributed through the hypoglossal nerve

## MULTIPLE CHOICE QUESTIONS

(Tick the single best correct option)

1. What is the procedure shown below?

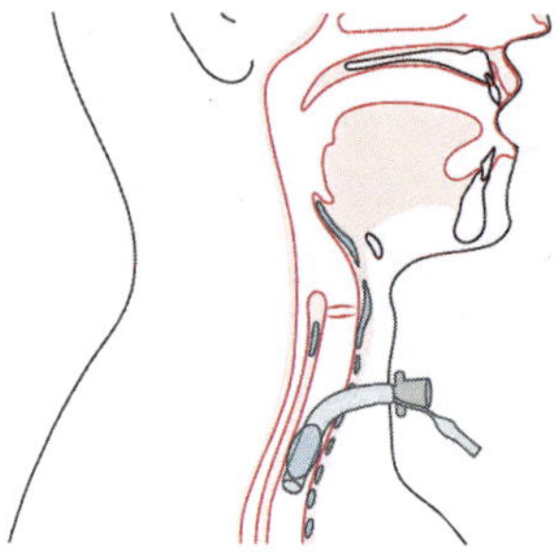

   a. Ryle's tube insertion  b. Thoracotomy
   c. Tracheostomy  d. Laryngoscopy

2. Adam's apple is formed by __________.
   a. Cricoid cartilage  b. Thyroid cartilage
   c. Aryepiglottic folds  d. Isthmus of thyroid gland

3. All of them are infrahyoid muscles, EXCEPT:
   a. Sternohyoid  b. Sternothyroid
   c. Thyrohyoid  d. Inferior belly of omohyoid

4. What is the nerve supply of thyrohyoid muscle?
   a. Ansa cervicalis
   b. Vagus nerve
   c. C1 via hypoglossal nerve
   d. External laryngeal nerve

5. The thyrohyoid membrane is pierced by __________.
   a. Internal laryngeal nerve
   b. External laryngeal nerve
   c. Recurrent laryngeal nerve
   d. Hypoglossal nerve

6. A 72-year-old male presented to the emergency department after experiencing a sudden episode of dizziness and loss of consciousness while turning his head to the left. After a few minutes he regained consciousness. What is the likely diagnosis?
   a. Orthostatic hypotension
   b. Carotid sinus syndrome
   c. Vasovagal syncope
   d. Cardiac arrhythmias

7. Ascending pharyngeal artery is a branch of __________.
   a. Superficial temporal artery
   b. Mandibular artery
   c. Maxillary artery
   d. External carotid artery

8. The second part of the lingual artery travels beneath __________ muscle.
   a. Geniohyoid
   b. Mylohyoid
   c. Hyoglossus
   d. Styloglossus

9. What is the significance of the carotid body?
   a. It regulates blood pressure by detecting changes in blood pressure levels
   b. It monitors blood oxygen levels and helps regulate respiratory rate
   c. It produces hormones that control heart rate
   d. It filters toxins from the blood before it reaches the brain

10. Maxillary artery and __________ are the terminal branches of the external carotid artery.
    a. Superior thyroid artery
    b. Ascending palatine artery
    c. Ascending pharyngeal artery
    d. Superficial temporal artery

11. The posterior belly of the digastric muscle is innervated by __________ nerve.
    a. V  b. VII
    c. IX  d. XI

12. __________ artery is the only medial branch of external carotid artery.
    a. Superior thyroid
    b. Lingual
    c. Facial
    d. Ascending pharyngeal

## QUESTION BANK

(Use separate copy to solve the following questions)

Q 1. Discuss the origin, course and branches of external carotid artery. Add a note on clinical anatomy of superior thyroid artery.

Q 2. Write a short notes on:
   a. Digastric muscle
   b. Boundaries and contents of carotid triangle.
   c. Boundaries and contents of digastric triangle.
   d. Branches of facial artery
   e. Lingual artery
   f. Ansa cervicalis

Q 3. Write the anatomical basis for:
   a. Carotid sinus syndrome

# 5

# Parotid Region

eSmartQuiz

## CLINICOANATOMICAL PROBLEM

### Clinical Case 1

A 45-year-old female presented with swelling and increasing pain exacerbated during meals. On examination, her right parotid gland was visibly swollen, tender to touch, and warm. She reported difficulty chewing due to worsening pain. Saliva production from the affected gland was reduced. A diagnosis of **acute parotitis** was made.

1. What is acute parotitis?
2. Why there was increased pain during meals in this case?
3. Why parotid swelling is painful?
4. What is the commonest cause of acute parotitis?

### *Explanation*

1. 

2. 

3. 

4. 

## PRACTICE FIGURES

(Label the practice figures)

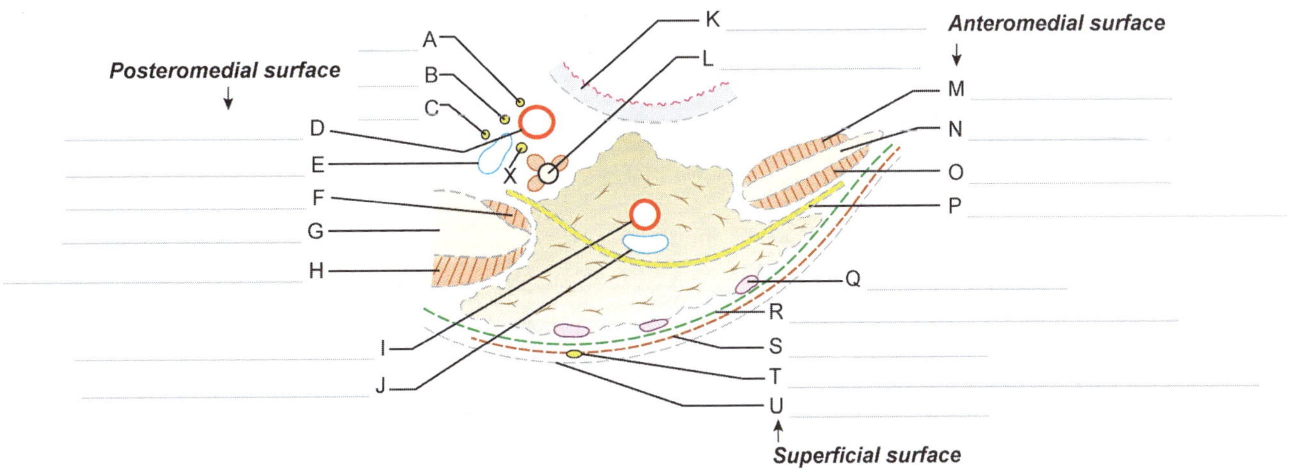


**Practice Figure 5.1:** Relations of the parotid gland

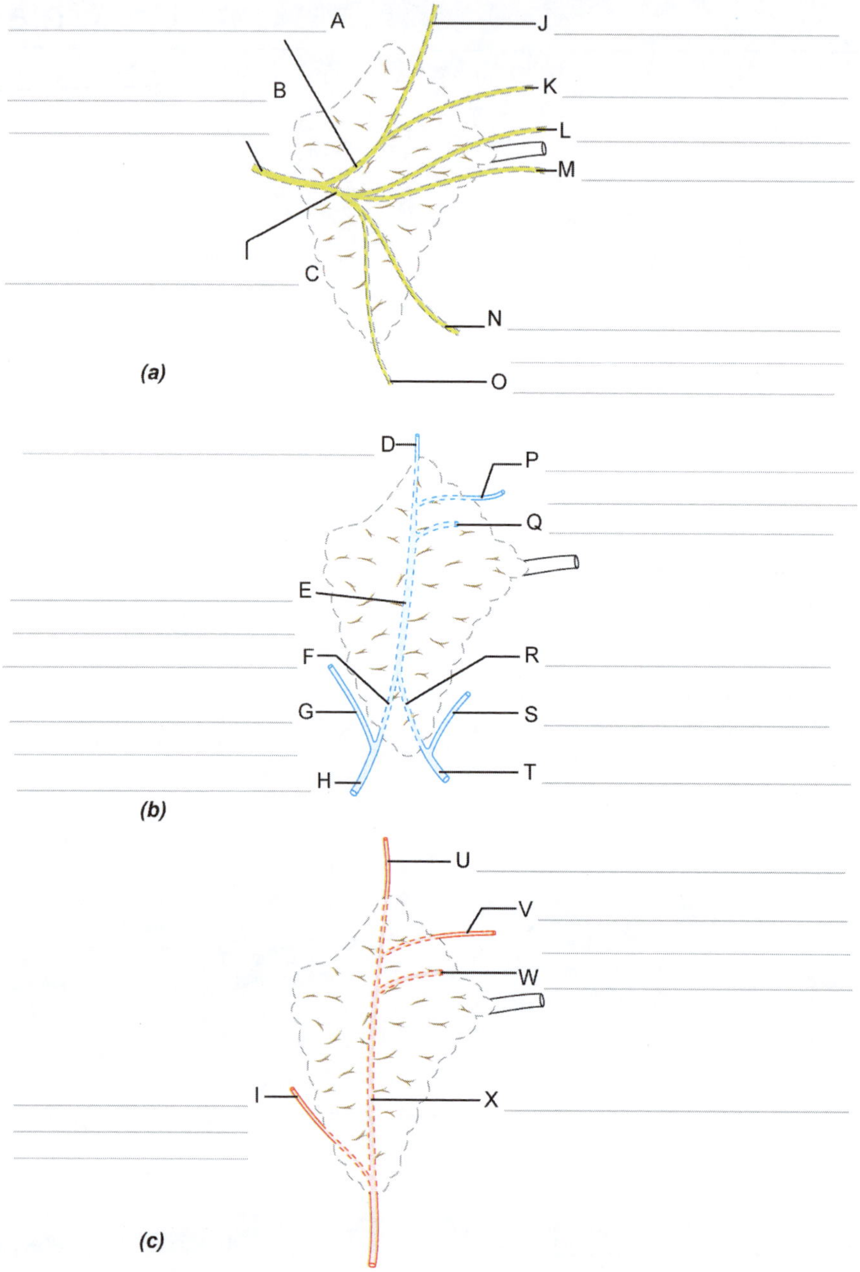


**Practice Figures 5.2a to c:** The structures traversing the parotid gland: (a) Facial nerve (pes anserinus branching pattern), (b) retromandibular vein, and (c) external carotid artery

## MULTIPLE CHOICE QUESTIONS

(Tick the single best correct option)

1. Stylomandibular ligament is pierced by ____________.
   a. Superficial temporal artery
   b. Facial artery
   c. External carotid artery
   d. Inferior alveolar artery
2. Which of the following statements is INCORRECT about the parotid gland?
   a. The investing layer of the deep cervical fascia forms a capsule for the gland.
   b. The apex of the gland is directed downwards.
   c. The external carotid artery enters the gland through the anteromedial surface.
   d. The retromandibular vein is formed within the gland by the union of the superficial temporal and maxillary veins.
3. From the picture, identify the nerve piercing the parotid parenchyma.

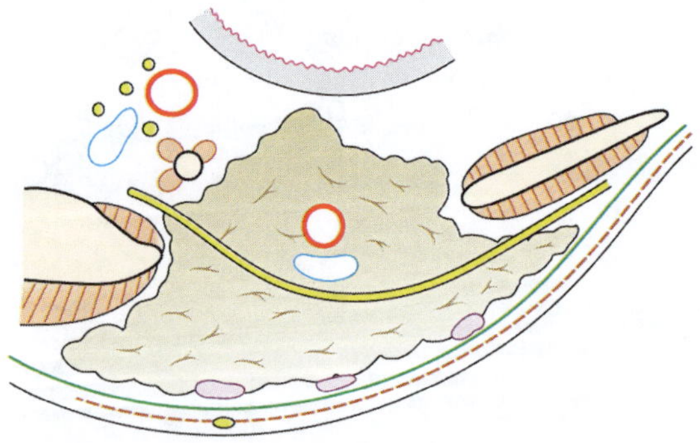

   a. Facial nerve
   b. Greater auricular nerve
   c. Auriculotemporal nerve
   d. Posterior auricular nerve

4. A 50-year-old female experiences sweating over the right side of the face while eating. She has undergone removal of right parotid gland six months back. What is the most likely diagnosis?
   a. Bell's palsy  b. Trigeminal neuralgia
   c. Frey's syndrome  d. Bell's palsy
5. Which salivary gland duct opens in the marked site?

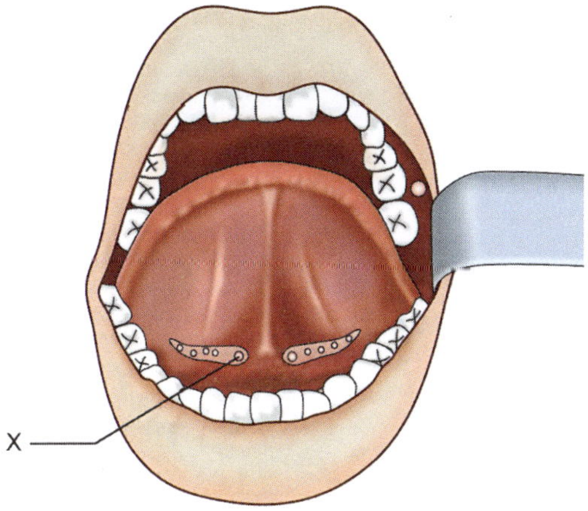


   a. Sublingual  b. Submandibular
   c. Parotid  d. Minor salivary gland
6. The secretomotor nerve supply of the parotid gland is carried by all of the following nerves, EXCEPT:
   a. Tympanic plexus  b. Glossopharyngeal nerve
   c. Lesser petrosal nerve  d. Mandibular nerve
7. Skin over the parotid gland is supplied by __________ nerve.
   a. Auriculotemporal  b. Facial
   c. Glossopharyngeal  d. Great auricular
8. Which procedure is used in draining parotid abscess?
   a. Marsupialization  b. Hilton's method
   c. Fistualisation  d. Sialadenectomy
9. From the image, name the vein marked as X?

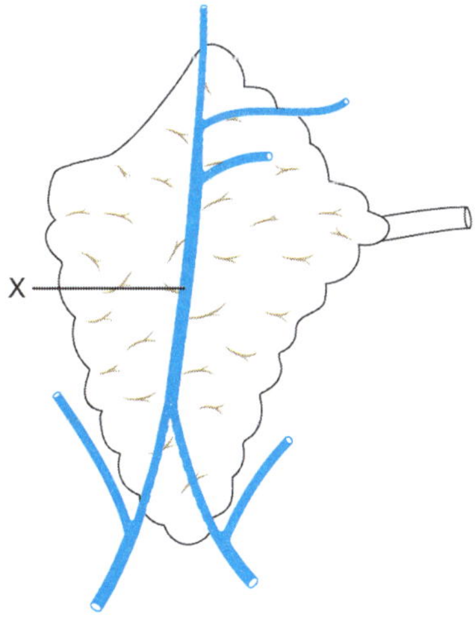


   a. External jugular vein  b. Facial vein
   c. Retromandibular vein  d. Posterior auricular vein
10. Stenson's duct opens into __________.
    a. The vestibule of the mouth
    b. Floor of mouth
    c. Circumvallate papillae
    d. Fungiform papillae
11. __________ artery passes between the roots of the auriculotemporal nerve.
    a. Maxillary
    b. Middle meningeal
    c. Superficial temporal
    d. Accessory meningeal
12. Pes anserinus arrangement is formed by __________ nerve.
    a. Oculomotor  b. Trigeminal
    c. Facial  d. Glossopharyngeal

## QUESTION BANK

(Use separate copy to solve the following questions)

Q 1. Describe the parotid gland under the following headings: Location, gross features, relations, blood supply, nerve supply and applied aspects.

Q 2. Describe the intraglandular structures of the parotid gland.

Q 3. Write a short notes on:
   a. Parotid duct
   b. Otic ganglion
   c. Capsule of parotid gland
   d. Facial nerve in the parotid gland

Q 4. Describe the anatomical basis of:
   a. Frey's syndrome
   b. Patey's faciovenous plane

Chapter

6

eSmartQuiz

# Temporal and Infratemporal Regions

## CLINICOANATOMICAL PROBLEMS

### Clinical Case 1

A 30-year-old male presented with sudden jaw pain and inability to open his mouth after yawning widely. On examination, his jaw was visibly deviated to one side, and attempts to open his mouth were met with resistance and severe pain. A diagnosis of **temporomandibular joint (TMJ) dislocation** was made. Immediate reduction was performed manually in the emergency department, resulting in relief of symptoms and restoration of normal jaw function.

1. Name the commonest type of TMJ dislocation.
2. Mention the site and direction of pressure to be applied during reduction of TMJ.

### Explanation

1. ______

2. ______

### Clinical Case 2

A 60-year-old chronic tobacco user male with a history of **cancer of tip of the tongue** presented with severe pain radiating to his left temporomandibular joint (TMJ), lower jaw, and temporal region.

1. Why is pain of tongue referred to lower jaw and TMJ?

### Explanation

1. ______

## PRACTICE FIGURES

(Label the practice figures)

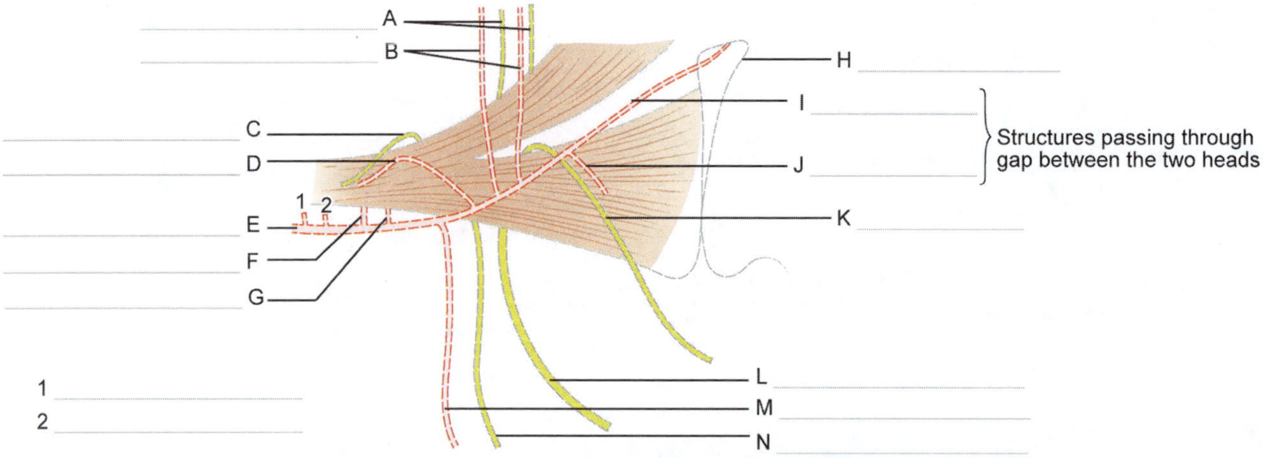


**Practice Figure 6.1:** Some relations of the lateral pterygoid muscle and branches of maxillary artery

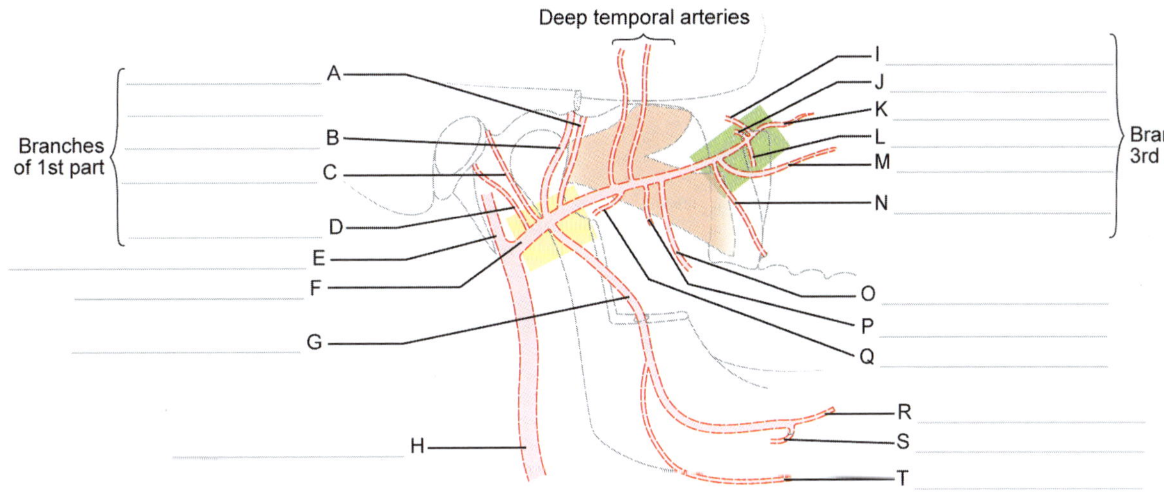


**Practice Figure 6.2:** Branches of three parts of the maxillary artery

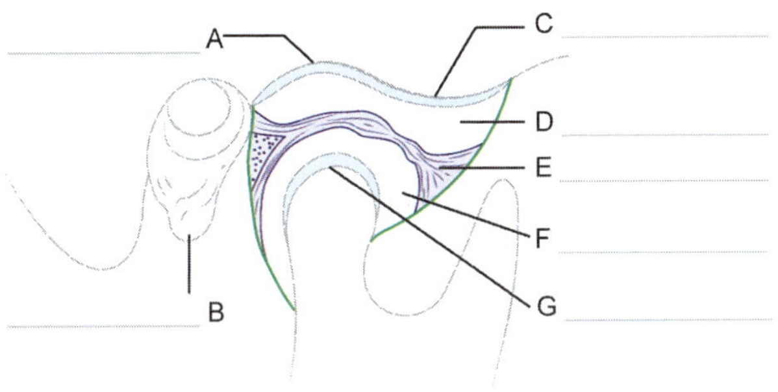


**Practice Figure 6.3:** Articular surfaces of right temporomandibular joint

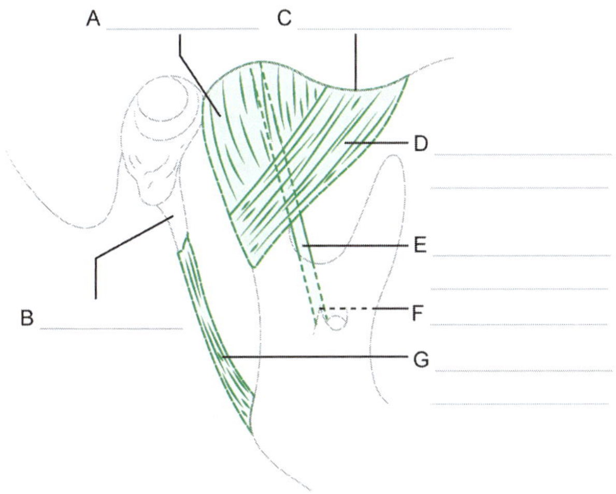


**Practice Figure 6.4:** Ligaments of the temporomandibular joint

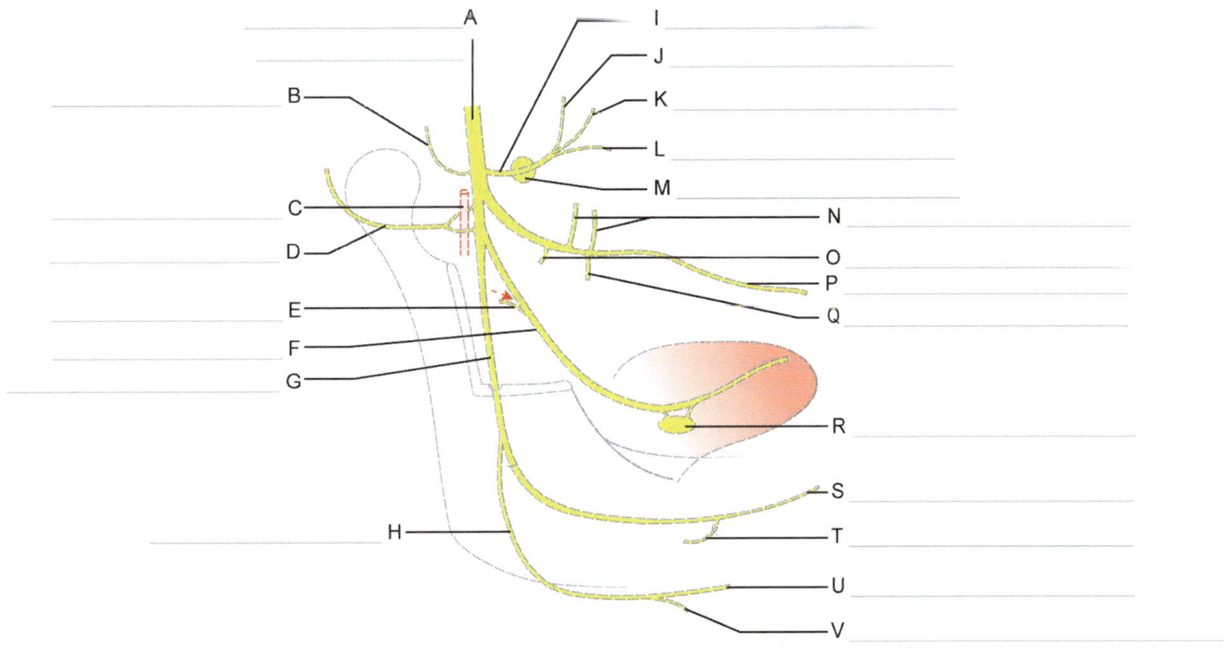


**Practice Figure 6.5:** Distribution of mandibular nerve (V3)

## MULTIPLE CHOICE QUESTIONS

(Tick the single best correct option)

1. Which of the following muscles helps in mastication?
   a. Lateral pterygoid  b. Buccinator
   c. Orbicularis oris  d. Hyoglossus
2. Which of the following structure emerges from the upper border of the lateral pterygoid muscle?
   a. Deep temporal nerve
   b. Maxillary artery
   c. Mandibular nerve
   d. Superficial temporal artery
3. A 25-year-old female went to a dental clinic with a history of dentine pain for 5 days. On examination, she had a malplaced wisdom tooth. Which nerve is likely to be injured while extracting the tooth?
   a. Buccal nerve
   b. Mandibular nerve
   c. Inferior alveolar nerve
   d. Lingual nerve
4. The articular surface of the temporomandibular joint is covered by ___________.
   a. Hyaline cartilage  b. Elastic cartilage
   c. Fibrocartilage  d. Capsular ligament
5. Identify the muscle marked by X in the following picture.

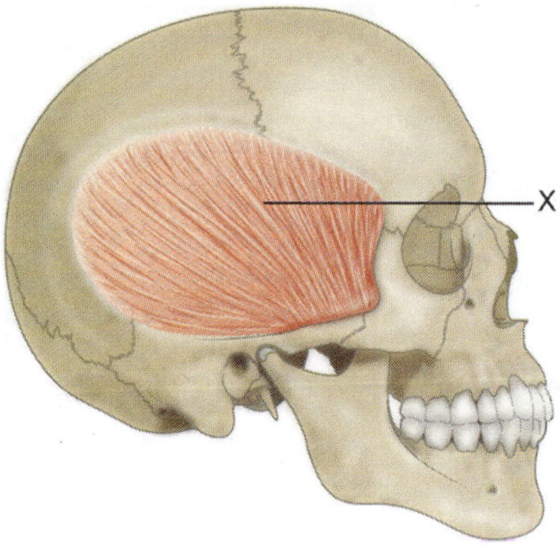


   a. Lateral pterygoid  b. Temporalis
   c. Masseter  d. Buccinator
6. Which nerve is infiltrated in the below shown image?

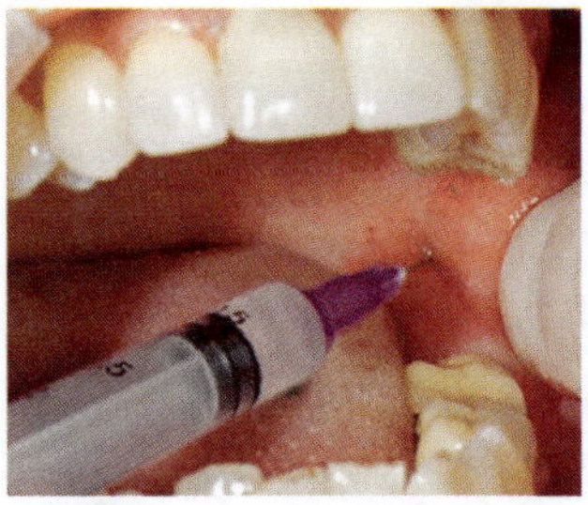

   a. Buccal nerve  b. Mandibular nerve
   c. Inferior alveolar nerve  d. Lingual nerve
7. Which is the only sensory branch of the anterior division of the mandibular nerve?
   a. Masseteric nerve
   b. Buccal nerve
   c. Auriculotemporal nerve
   d. Lingual nerve
8. Which of the following arteries is known as the artery of epistaxis?
   a. Deep temporal artery
   b. Artery of pterygoid canal
   c. Sphenopalatine artery
   d. Lesser palatine artery
9. Which among the following is NOT a branch of the 3rd part of the maxillary artery?
   a. Infraorbital artery
   b. Deep temporal artery
   c. Sphenopalatine artery
   d. Greater palatine artery
10. What is the significance of anteroinferior angle of the nasal septum?
    a. Vessels drain into cavernous sinus
    b. Presence of Kisesselbach's plexus
    c. More prone for fracture
    d. Rich nerve supply
11. Structures emerging at the lower border of lateral pterygoid are all, EXCEPT:
    a. Deep temporal nerves
    b. Lingual nerve
    c. Middle meningeal artery
    d. Inferior alveolar nerve and artery

## QUESTION BANK

(Use separate copy to solve the following questions)

Q 1. Describe the muscles of mastication under the following headings: Origin, insertion, nerve supply, actions, and applied aspects.

Q 2. Describe the temporomandibular joint under the following headings: Type of joint, articular surfaces, ligaments, relations, movements, applied aspects.

Q 3. Describe the maxillary artery under the following headings: Beginning, course, termination, relations, branches, and applied aspects.

Q 4. Write a short notes on:
   a. Relations of lateral pterygoid muscle
   b. Otic ganglion
   c. Mandibular nerve
   d. Branches of maxillary artery
   e. Sphenomandibular ligament
   f. Factors maintaining stability of temporomandibular joint.

Q 5. Explain the anatomical basis for:
   a. Reduction of dislocated TMJ
   b. Clicking sound at TMJ

Chapter

7

# Submandibular Region

eSmartQuiz

## CLINICOANATOMICAL PROBLEM

### Clinical Case 1

A 55-year-old male presented with swelling and pain under his jaw, worsening during meals. On examination, a firm, tender mass was palpated in the submandibular region. Bimanual palpation revealed a hard stone within the duct of the submandibular gland. CT scan confirmed the presence of a salivary duct stone.

1. Why there was increased pain during meals?
2. Why is bimanual palpation needed for the submandibular gland?
3. What is sialography?

### Explanation

1. ______

2. ______

3. ______

## PRACTICE FIGURES

(Label the practice figures)

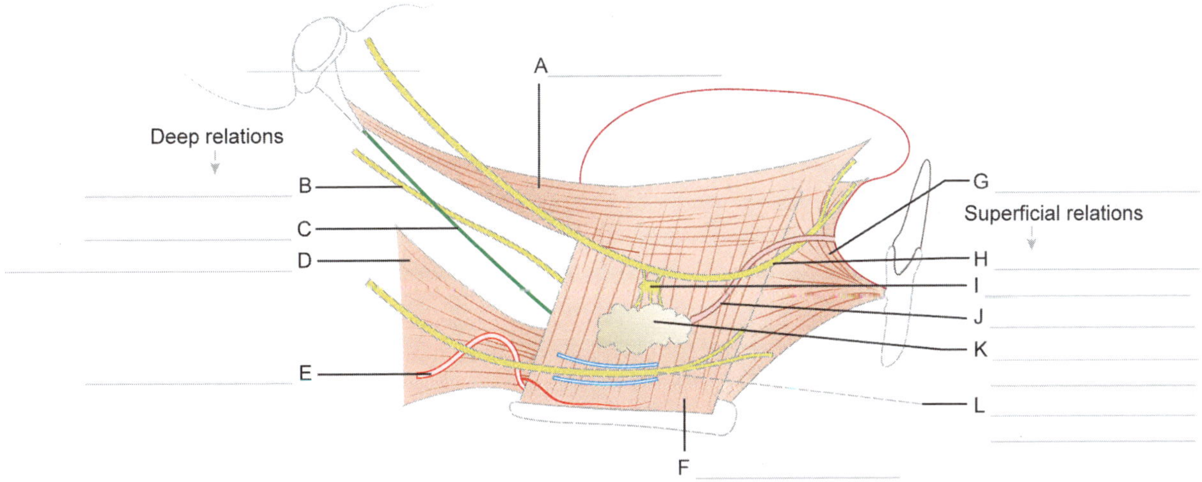


**Practice Figure 7.1:** Relations of the hyoglossus muscle

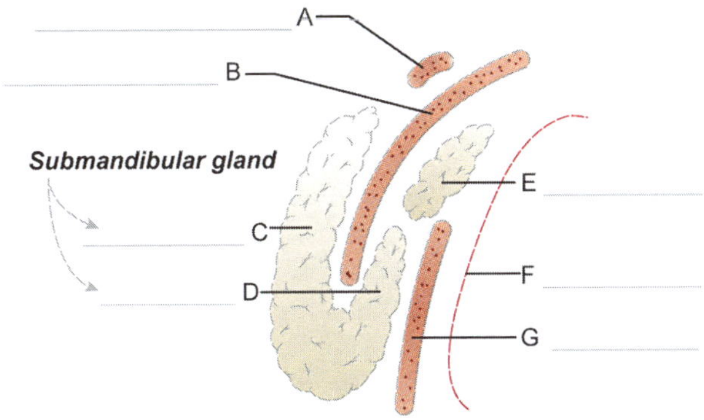


**Practice Figure 7.2:** Location of the submandibular and sublingual glands

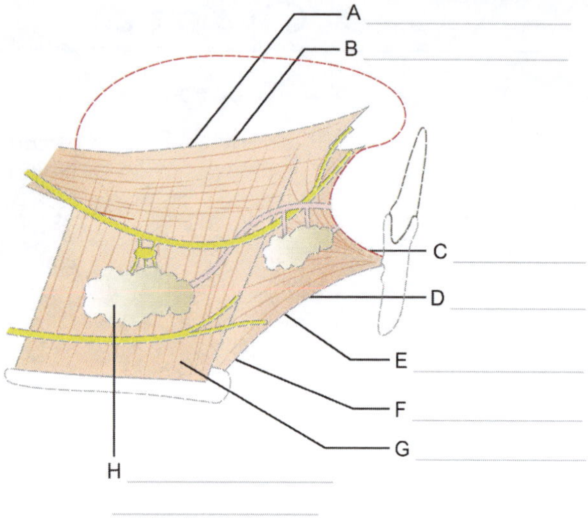


**Practice Figure 7.3:** Deep part of submandibular gland and sublingual gland

## MULTIPLE CHOICE QUESTIONS

(Tick the single best correct option)

1. Taste from the circumvallate papillae is carried by ___________.
   a. Chorda tympani nerve
   b. Hypoglossal nerve
   c. Glossopharyngeal nerve.
   d. Vagus nerve
2. Posterior belly of digastric muscle is supplied by ___________.
   a. Facial nerve
   b. Nerve to mylohyoid
   c. Chorda tympani nerve
   d. Hypoglossal nerve
3. Name the muscles marked with X that divides the submandibular gland into two halves.

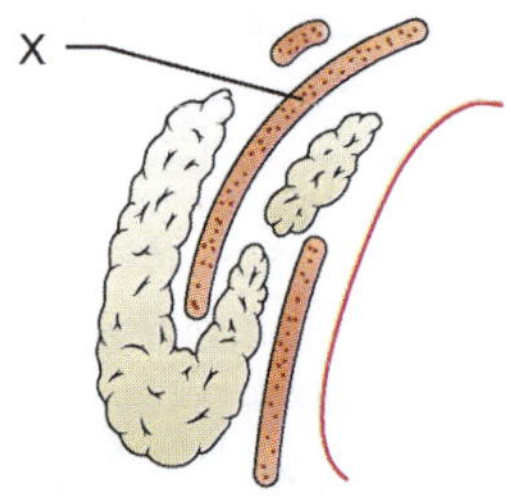


   a. Hyoglossus b. Genioglossus
   c. Mylohyoid d. Masseter
4. Which is known as the chief artery of palatine tonsil?
   a. Facial artery
   b. Ascending pharyngeal artery
   c. Ascending palatine artery
   d. Lingual artery
5. Which of the following nerve supply the anterior two-thirds of the tongue?
   a. Chorda tympani nerve
   b. Spinal accessory nerve
   c. Glossopharyngeal nerve
   d. Vagus nerve
6. A 45-year-old male presented to the dental clinic with complaints of recurrent pain and swelling in the right side of his lower jaw. The pain increases during meals and gradually decreases. He also reported a dry mouth and difficulty swallowing. Which of the following is the most likely cause of the patient's symptoms?
   a. Temporomandibular joint disorder
   b. Submandibular duct stone
   c. Dental abscess
   d. Mumps
7. Which salivary gland is examined in the image shown below?

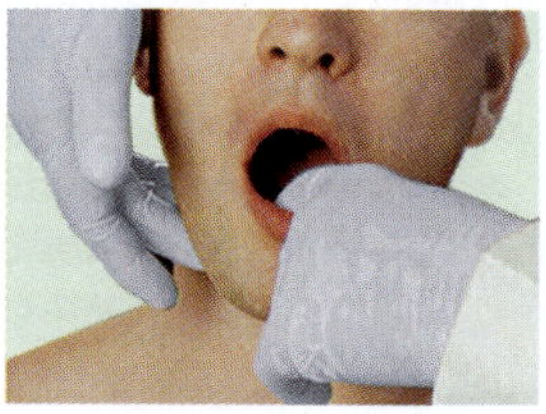

   a. Sublingual b. Minor salivary
   c. Parotid d. Submandibular
8. Stylohyoid is innervated by ___________.
   a. IX b. X
   c. VII d. VIII
9. Which among the following is known as a life-saving muscle?
   a. Hyoglossus
   b. Genioglossus
   c. Geniohyoid
   d. Mylohyoid
10. Which type of secretion is primarily produced by the submandibular gland under parasympathetic stimulation?
    a. Mucous
    b. Serous
    c. Seromucinous
    d. Watery

## QUESTION BANK

(Use separate copy to solve the following questions)

Q 1. Describe the submandibular gland under the following headings: Features, coverings, relations, duct, nerve supply, and applied aspects.

Q 2. Write a short notes on:
   a. Digastric muscle
   b. Hyoglossus muscle
   c. Submandibular ganglion.

eSmartQuiz

# Structures in the Neck

## CLINICOANATOMICAL PROBLEM

### Clinical Case 1

A 50-year-old female presented with progressively enlarging neck swelling and hoarseness of voice over several months. On examination, a firm, enlarged thyroid gland was noted, moving with deglutition. The patient reported difficulty swallowing and a change in her voice. Ultrasound confirmed a multinodular goitre. Fine needle aspiration biopsy was performed to rule out malignancy.

1. What is goitre?
2. Why does thyroid swelling move with deglutition?
3. Why there is hoarseness of voice in this case?

*Explanation*

1. ______________________

2. ______________________

3. ______________________

## PRACTICE FIGURES

(Label the practice figures)

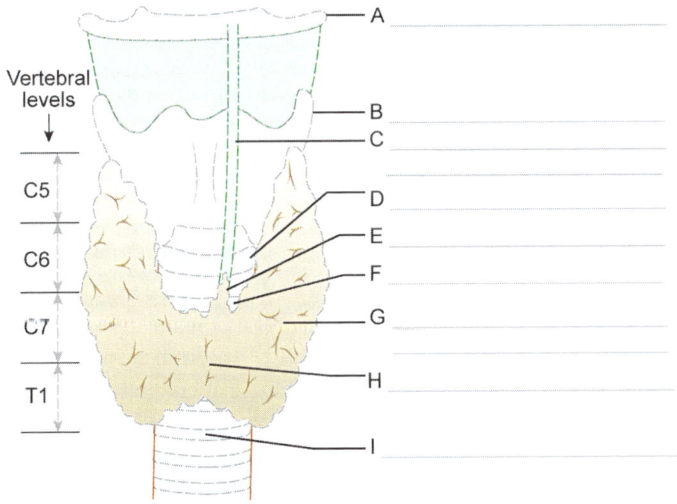


**Practice Figure 8.1:** Parts and extent of the thyroid gland

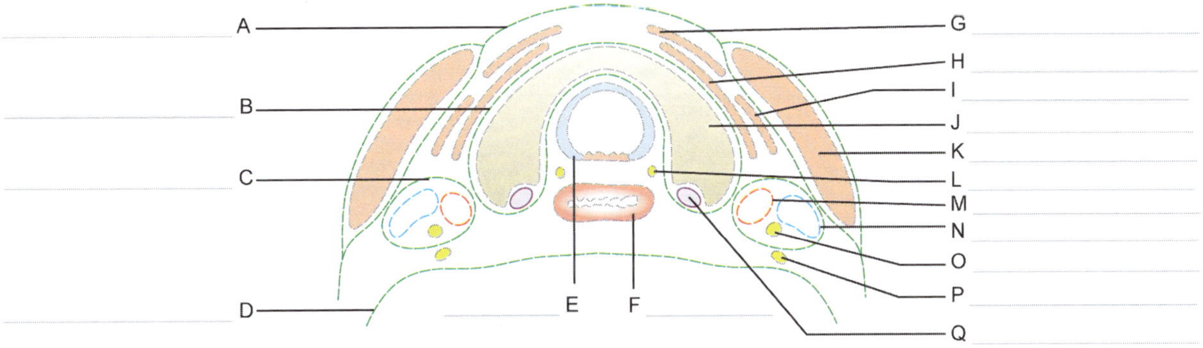


**Practice Figure 8.2:** Relations of thyroid gland

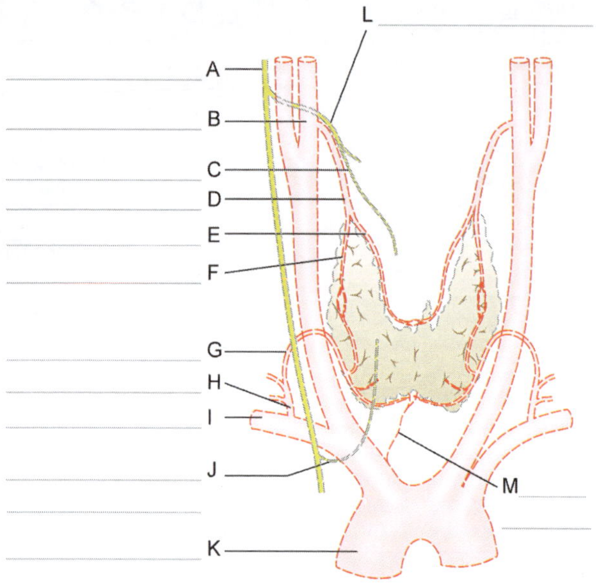


Practice Figure 8.3: Arterial supply of thyroid gland

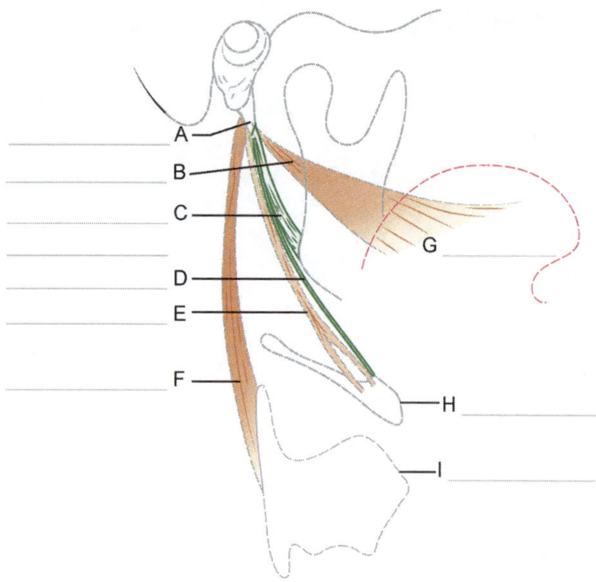


Practice Figure 8.4: Styloid apparatus

## MULTIPLE CHOICE QUESTIONS

(Tick the single best correct option)

1. Which structure prevents thyroid from descending down?
   a. Hyoid bone
   b. Thyrohyoid membrane
   c. Ligament of Berry
   d. Cricothyroid ligament
2. The superior thyroid artery is accompanied by ________.
   a. Recurrent laryngeal nerve
   b. External laryngeal nerve
   c. Internal laryngeal nerve
   d. Vagus nerve
3. The structure marked by X is the remnant of ________.

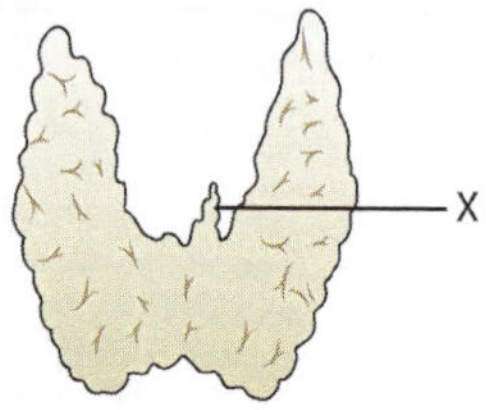


   a. Thyroid cartilage
   b. Thyroglossal duct
   c. Isthmus
   d. Cricoid cartilage
4. From the below image identify the structure marked as X which divides the subclavian artery into three parts?

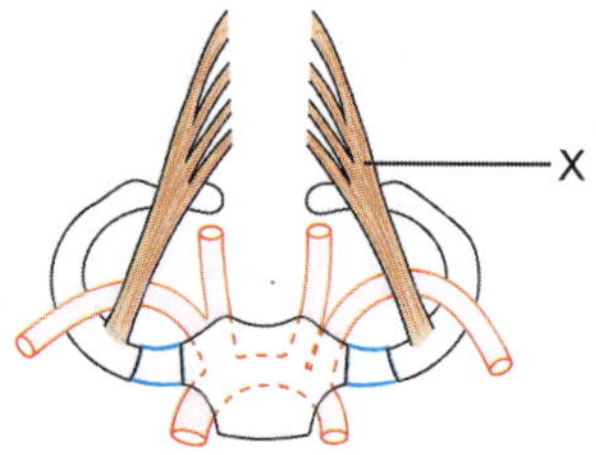


   a. Scalenus medius
   b. Scalenus anterior
   c. Scalenus posterior muscle
   d. Sternocleidomastoid muscle
5. A 48-year-old woman underwent a total thyroidectomy for the multinodular goitre. The surgery was uneventful, and she was discharged the next day. Two days after the surgery, she had tingling sensations around her mouth and in her fingers and toes. She also noticed muscle cramps and spasms in her hands. What could be the likely cause?
   a. Hypocalcemia due to accidental removal of the parathyroid glands
   b. Hyperthyroidism due to inadequate thyroidectomy
   c. Hypokalemia due to fluid imbalance
   d. Infection at the surgical site
6. The inferior thyroid artery is a branch of ________.
   a. Internal carotid artery
   b. Subclavian artery
   c. External carotid artery
   d. Thyrocervical trunk
7. Which of the following statements is true regarding Kocher's vein?
   a. It drains directly into the subclavian vein.
   b. It drains into the internal jugular vein.
   c. It originates from the lower pole of the thyroid gland.
   d. It is also known as the inferior thyroid vein.
8. Dorsal scapular artery is a branch of ________.
   a. First part of subclavian
   b. Second part of subclavian
   c. Third part of subclavian
   d. Thyrocervical trunk
9. Which is the main node draining the tonsil?
   a. Jugulo omohyoid
   b. Jugulodigastric
   c. Submandibular
   d. Sublingual

10. Which of the following is not a feature of Horner's syndrome?
    a. Exophthalmos
    b. Ptosis
    c. Loss of the ciliospinal reflex
    d. Anhidrosis
11. Hoarseness of voice is seen after thyroidectomy due to injury of __________ nerve.
    a. Superior laryngeal
    b. Phrenic
    c. Recurrent laryngeal
    d. Internal laryngeal
12. All of the following muscles are supplied by the ansa cervicalis, EXCEPT:
    a. Sternohyoid
    b. Sternothyroid
    c. Geniohyoid
    d. Inferior belly of omohyoid

## QUESTION BANK

(Use separate copy to solve the following questions)

Q 1. Describe the thyroid gland under the following headings: Gross features, relations, blood supply, applied aspects.

Q 2. Write a short notes on:
   a. Capsule of thyroid gland
   b. Blood supply of thyroid gland
   c. Name the branches of subclavian artery
   d. Branches of subclavian artery
   e. Branches of internal carotid artery
   f. Tributaries of internal jugular vein
   g. Styloid apparatus

Q 3. Describe the anatomical basis of:
   a. Horner's syndrome
   b. Subclavian steal syndrome
   c. Queckenstedt's test.

Chapter

9

eSmartQuiz

# Prevertebral and Paravertebral Regions

## CLINICOANATOMICAL PROBLEMS

### Clinical Case 1

A 40-year-old male died in a car accident after his vehicle was rear-ended. The car seat was faulty, lacking a headrest. Post-mortem examination revealed a **fracture of the odontoid process** of the C2 vertebra, leading to fatal spinal cord injury.

1. Why the odontoid process fracture lead to death in this case?
2. Why does the headrest is important in car?
3. Name the ligaments attached to the odontoid process.

#### *Explanation*

1. ______________________________

2. ______________________________

3. ______________________________

### Clinical Case 2

A 62-year-old male with a history of smoking presented with progressive dysphagia, initially to solids and later to liquids. He developed hoarseness of voice and noticeable weight loss over three months. Examination revealed cervical lymphadenopathy. Endoscopy confirmed a diagnosis of **carcinoma of the oesophagus**. The patient underwent a biopsy, which revealed squamous cell carcinoma.

1. Why did the patient have dysphagia in this case?
2. Name the deep cervical nodes.
3. Why did the patient have hoarseness of voice in this case?

#### *Explanation*

1. ______________________________

2. ______________________________

3. ______________________________

## PRACTICE FIGURES

(Label the practice figures)

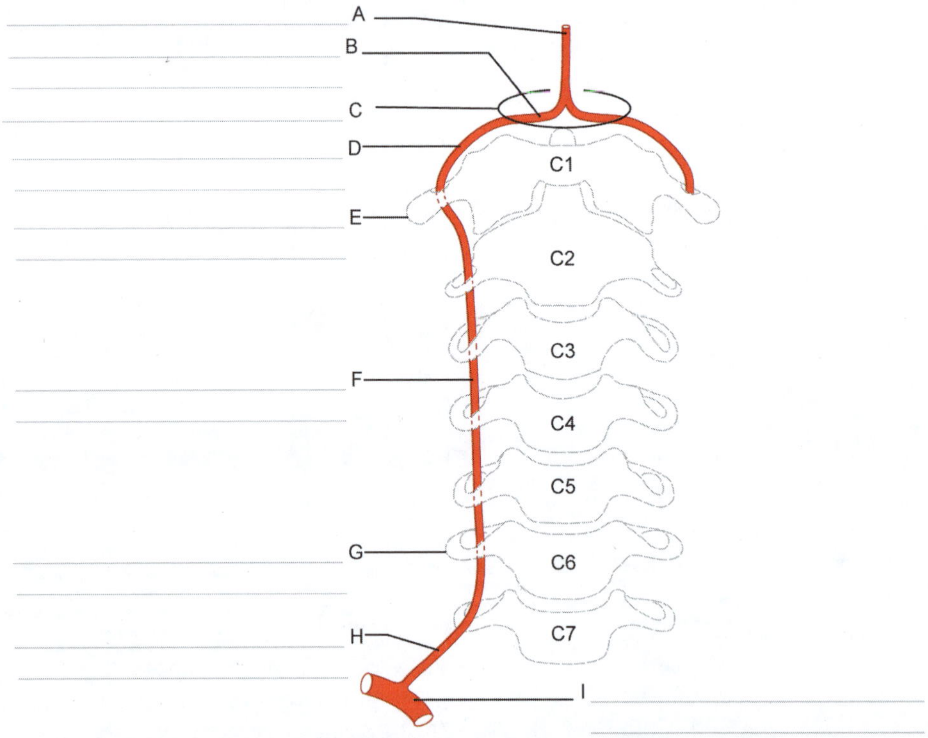


**Practice Figure 9.1:** Vertebral artery

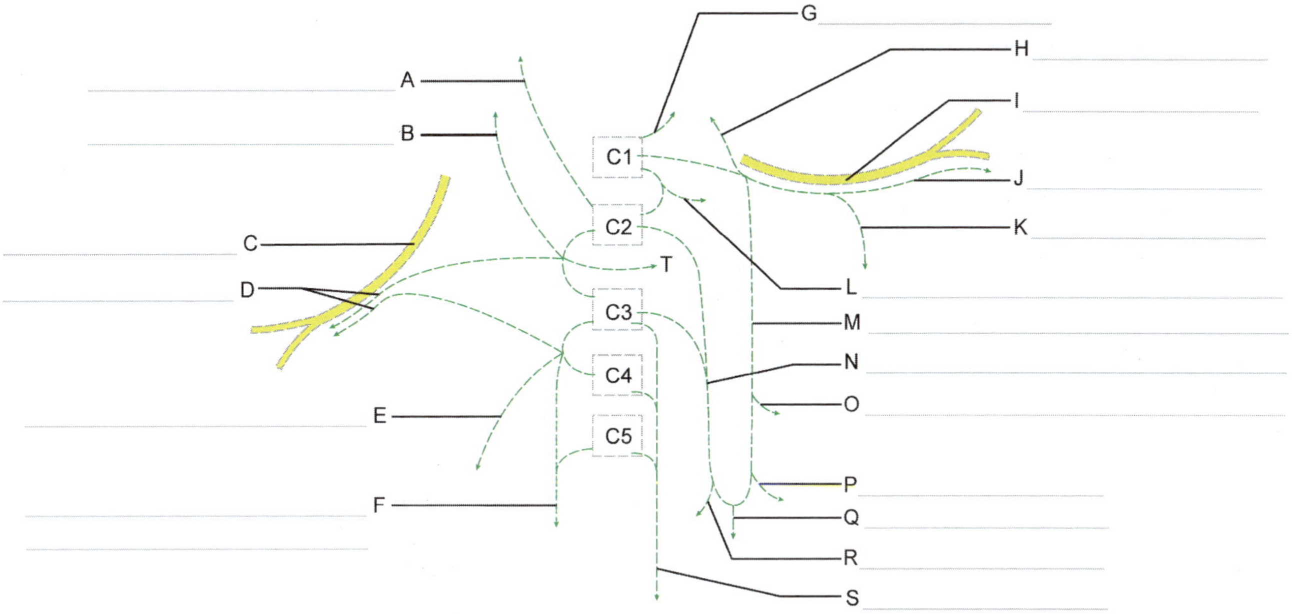


**Practice Figure 9.2:** Cervical plexus and its branches (T: transverse cutaneous nerve of neck [C2, C3]

## MULTIPLE CHOICE QUESTIONS

(Tick the single best correct option)

1. What is the content of the scalenovertebral triangle?
   a. Scalenus anterior
   b. Transverse process of C6 vertebra
   c. First part of vertebral artery
   d. Cervical part of parasympathetic trunk
2. Trachea begins at the level of ____________.
   a. Lower border of C6 vertebra
   b. Lower border of C5 vertebra
   c. Lower border of C7 vertebra
   d. Lower border of C4 vertebra
3. Which structure is retracted during tracheostomy procedure?
   a. Right lobe of thyroid  b. Left lobe of thyroid
   c. Isthmus  d. Pyramidal lobe
4. Name the structure marked by X in the following picture.

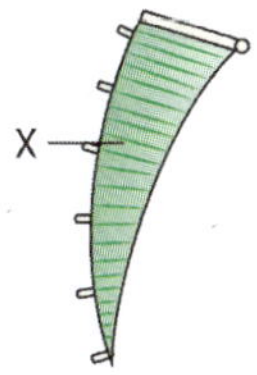


   a. Anterior longitudinal ligament
   b. Posterior longitudinal ligament
   c. Ligament of dens
   d. Ligamentum nuchae
5. Turning of head from side-to-side is caused at __________ joint.
   a. Atlantoaxial  b. Atlanto-occipital
   c. Zygapophyseal  d. Intervertebral
6. A 38-year-old IT employee came with a history of chronic neck pain that has progressively worsened over the past one year. He also reports occasional numbness and tingling in his right arm and hand. What is the possible cause?
   a. Cervical rib
   b. Cervical spondylosis with radiculopathy
   c. Intervertebral disc prolapse
   d. Atlantoaxial joint dislocation
7. What type of joint is formed between the dens of the axis and the atlas?
   a. Hinge  b. Pivot
   c. Saddle  d. Condyloid
8. Identify the nerve marked as X in the below image.

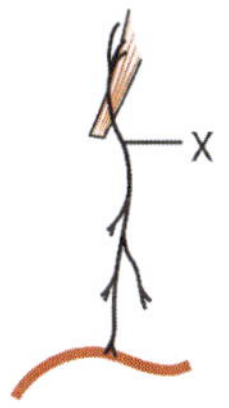


   a. Phrenic  b. Ansa cervicalis
   c. Vagus  d. Cervical sympathetic trunk
9. Scalenus minimus is the expansion of ____________.
   a. Scalenus anterior  b. Scalenus medius
   c. Suprapleural membrane  d. Scalenus posterior
10. The notochord continues as ____________.
    a. Membrana tectoria  b. Cruciate ligament
    c. Alar ligament  d. Apical ligament of dens
11. The membrana tectoria is the upward continuation of ____________ ligament.
    a. Posterior longitudinal  b. Ligamentum nuchae
    c. Ligamentum flava  d. Anterior longitudinal

## QUESTION BANK

(Use separate copy to solve the following questions)

Q 1. Write a short notes on:
   a. Vertebral artery
   b. Atlantoaxial joint
   c. Atlanto-occipital joint
   d. Constriction of oesophagus
   e. Contents of scalenovertebral angle

Q 2. Write the anatomical basis for:
   a. Death in judicial hanging

Chapter

# 10

eSmartQuiz

# Back of the Neck

## CLINICOANATOMICAL PROBLEM

### Clinical Case 1

A 8-year-old girl presented with a **sore throat**, difficulty drinking water, and neck stiffness over a week. She also reported a severe headache that worsened over time. Examination revealed nuchal rigidity and fever. Lumbar puncture confirmed a diagnosis of bacterial **meningitis**.

1. What is sore throat?
2. How did the sore throat turn into meningitis?
3. Why is there neck stiffness in meningitis?
4. What is the site of CSF collection in the neck?

### *Explanation*

1. ______________________________

2. ______________________________

3. ______________________________

4. ______________________________

## PRACTICE FIGURE

(Label the practice figure)

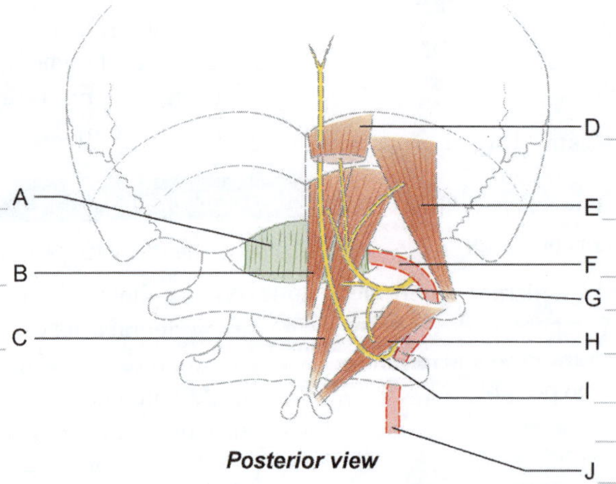


**Practice Figure 10.1:** Suboccipital triangle

## MULTIPLE CHOICE QUESTIONS

(Tick the single best correct option)

1. Which of the following is the thickest cutaneous nerve in the body?
   a. Greater occipital nerve b. Third occipital nerve
   c. Greater auricular nerve d. Lesser occipital nerve
2. Deep cervical artery is a branch of __________.
   a. Brachiocephalic trunk b. Occipital artery
   c. Subclavian artery d. Vertebral artery
3. For which condition, the following test is performed?

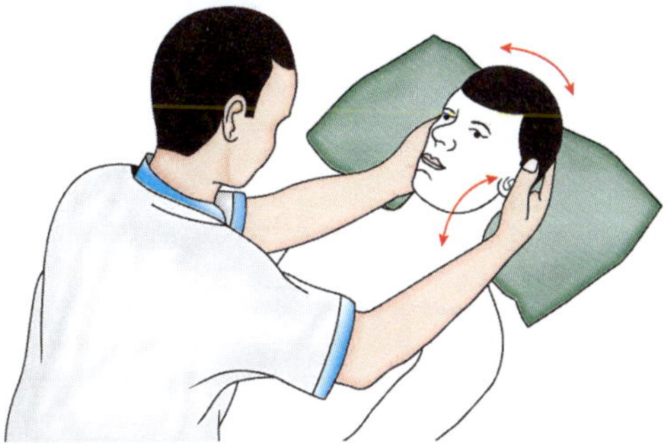

   a. Cervical spondylosis b. Spinal cord injury
   c. Meningitis d. Cervical rib
4. Which part of the vertebral artery passes through the suboccipital triangle?
   a. 1st part b. 2nd part
   c. 4th part d. 3rd part
5. What is the nerve supply of the marked muscle with X?

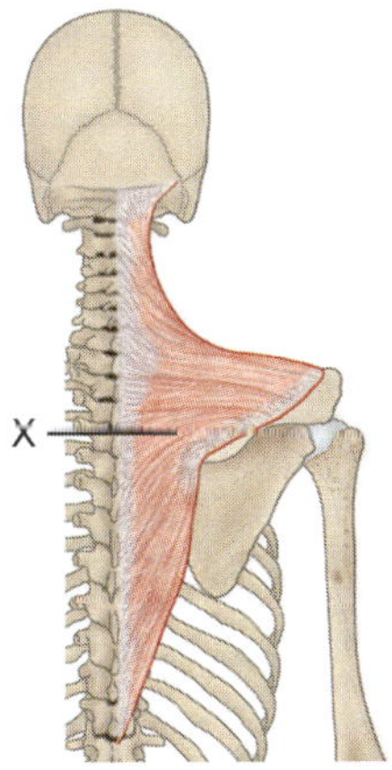


   a. Axillary nerve b. Spinal accessory nerve
   c. Dorsal scapular nerve d. Long thoracic nerve
6. The inferior thyroid artery is a branch of __________.
   a. Internal carotid artery
   b. Subclavian artery
   c. External carotid artery
   d. Thyrocervical trunk
7. What is the cutaneous nerve supply of the nape of neck?
   a. Greater occipital nerve
   b. Lesser occipital nerve
   c. Great auricular nerve
   d. Supraclavicular nerve
8. All the suboccipital muscles are supplied by:
   a. C1 dorsal ramus b. C2 dorsal ramus
   c. C3 dorsal ramus d. C4 dorsal ramus
9. The part of the vertebral artery that lies in the vertebral canal is:
   a. First part b. Second part
   c. Third part d. Fourth part
10. Which of the following is the climbing muscle?
    a. Trapezius b. Latissimus dorsi
    c. Levator scapulae d. Rhomboid major

## QUESTION BANK

(Use separate copy to solve the following question)

Q 1. Write a short notes on:
   a. Boundaries and contents of suboccipital triangle
   b. Occipital artery
   c. Suboccipital nerve.

Chapter

# 11

# Contents of Vertebral Canal

eSmartQuiz

## CLINICOANATOMICAL PROBLEM

### Clinical Case 1

A 70-year-old male with a history of **prostate cancer** presented with worsening back pain and neurological deficits. MRI revealed metastases to the cervical vertebrae and brain.

1. How the cancer cells from the prostate spread to the brain.

### *Explanation*

1. ____________________

## PRACTICE FIGURES

(Label the practice figures)

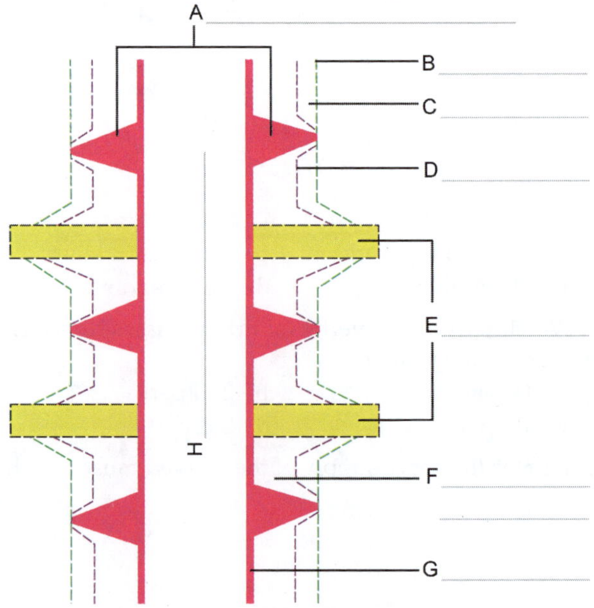


**Practice Figure 11.1:** Ligamentum denticulatum and its relationship to the dura mater and to the arachnoid mater

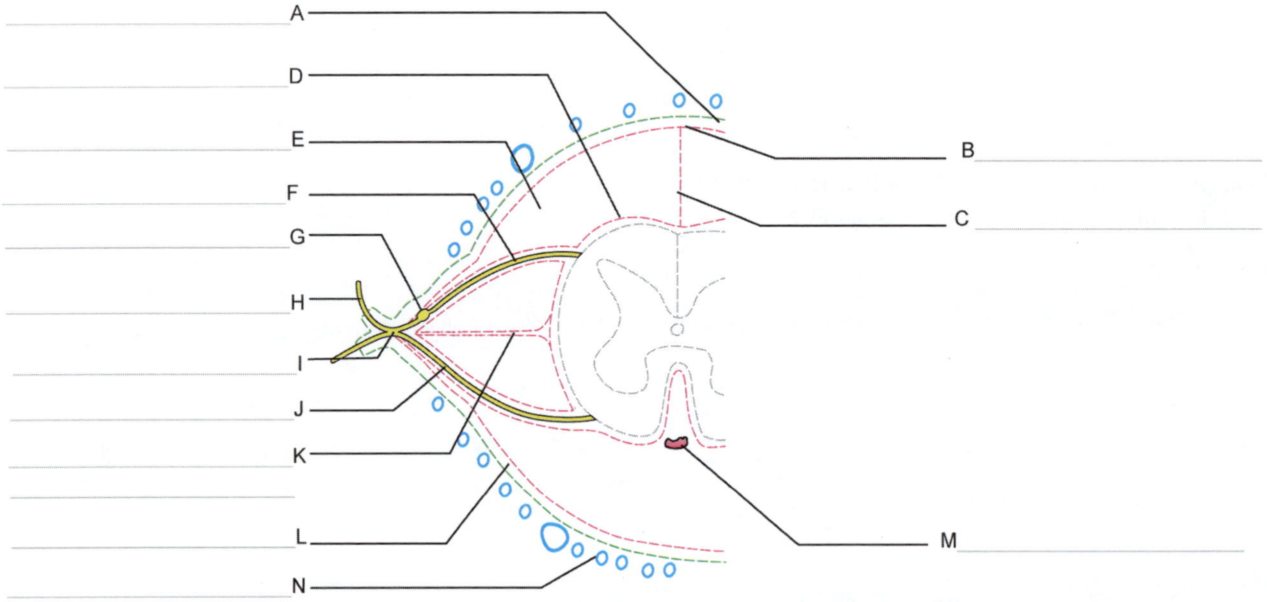


**Practice Figure 11.2:** Schematic transverse section showing the spinal meninges

## MULTIPLE CHOICE QUESTIONS

(Tick the single best correct option)

1. At which site is a lumbar puncture typically performed?
   a. Between L2 and L3
   b. Between L1 and L2
   c. Between L3 and L4
   d. Between S1 and S2
2. Which of the following is NOT a content of the epidural space?
   a. Loose areolar tissue b. Semiliquid fat
   c. Spinal arteries d. Meningeal artery
3. Which of the following is NOT true about spinal dura mater?
   a. It is a thick, tough fibrous membrane around the spinal cord.
   b. It is continuous with the meningeal layer of the cerebral dura mater.
   c. It extends from the foramen magnum to the lower border of the third sacral vertebra.
   d. It gives tubular prolongations to the dorsal and ventral nerve roots.
4. Where is the subarachnoid space located?
   a. Between the dura mater and the skull
   b. Between the pia mater and the brain
   c. Between the arachnoid mater and the dura mater
   d. Between the pia mater and the arachnoid mater
5. What structure passes through the site marked as X?

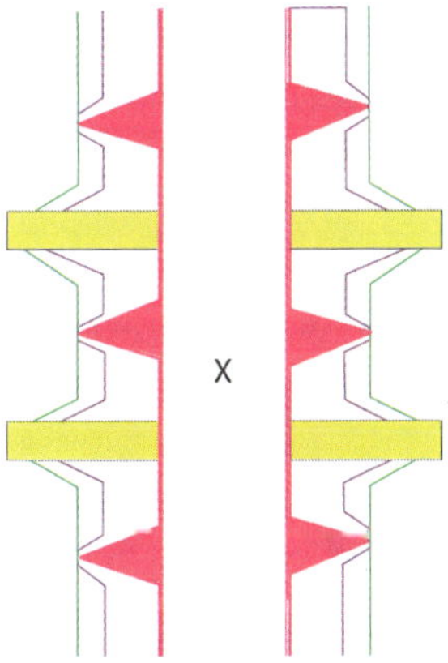


   a. Spinal cord b. Dorsal ramus
   c. Ventral ramus d. Vertebral artery
6. Which of the following cancers produce secondaries to the cranial cavity via vertebral venous plexus?
   a. Carcinoma of stomach b. Carcinoma of prostate
   c. Carcinoma of colon d. Carcinoma of ovary
7. A 52-year-old warehouse worker presented with sudden severe lower back pain radiating to both legs, saddle anaesthesia, urinary incontinence, and leg weakness. What is your probable diagnosis based on the history?
   a. Multiple sclerosis
   b. Conus medullaris syndrome
   c. Cauda equina syndrome
   d. Spinal haematoma
8. Identify the space marked as X in the below image.

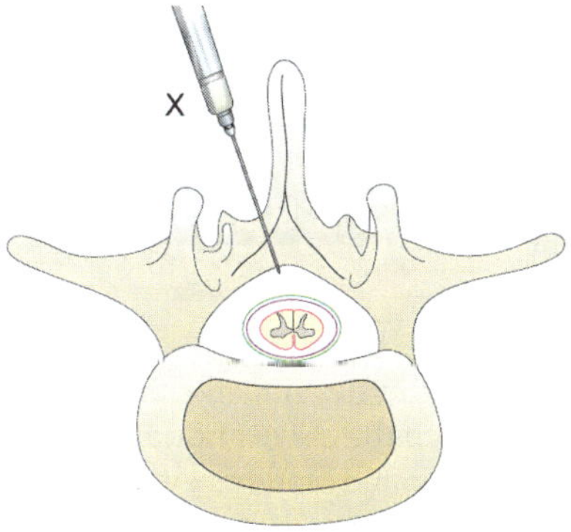


   a. Subdural space b. Subarachnoid space
   c. Epidural space d. Extradural space
9. What are leptomeninges?
   a. Dura mater and arachnoid mater
   b. Pia mater and dura mater
   c. Arachnoid mater and pia mater
   d. Dura mater only
10. Identify the true statement about the spinal nerves from the following statements:
    a. The spinal cord gives rise to 31 pairs of spinal nerves
    b. The spinal nerve has two roots—ventral sensory and dorsal motor
    c. The roots of spinal nerves are surrounded by sheaths derived from the meninges
    d. Below the lower end of the spinal cord, the roots form a bundle known as the cauda equina
11. Subarachnoid space extends up to the ___________ vertebra.
    a. S1 b. S2
    c. L1 d. L3

## QUESTION BANK

(Use separate copy to solve the following question)

Q 1. Write a short notes on:
   a. Contents of vertebral canal
   b. Epidural space
   c. Ligamentum dentaticulum and its surgical importance
   d. Batson venous plexus

# Chapter 12

eSmartQuiz

# Cranial Cavity

## CLINICOANATOMICAL PROBLEMS

### Clinical Case 1

A 40-year-old contractor sustained a severe head injury at work. Subsequently, he developed pulsating exophthalmos and a protruded eyeball. On examination, his conjunctival blood vessels were dilated, and his eyeball pulsated with his arterial pulse. He complained of a rumbling sound in the orbit and experienced venous congestion and impaired vision. The diagnosis was a carotid-cavernous fistula, resulting from the head trauma.

1. What is carotid-cavernous fistula?
2. Why was there an pulsating exophthalmos?

### Explanation

1. ______________________________

2. ______________________________

### Clinical Case 2

A 45-year-old woman experienced gradual loss of peripheral vision, leading to bitemporal hemianopia and tubular vision. She reported frequent headaches and fatigue. An MRI revealed a pituitary tumour.

1. Why was there a bitemporal hemianopia?
2. Why was there a tubular vision?

### Explanation

1. ______________________________

2. ______________________________

## PRACTICE FIGURES

(Label the practice figures)

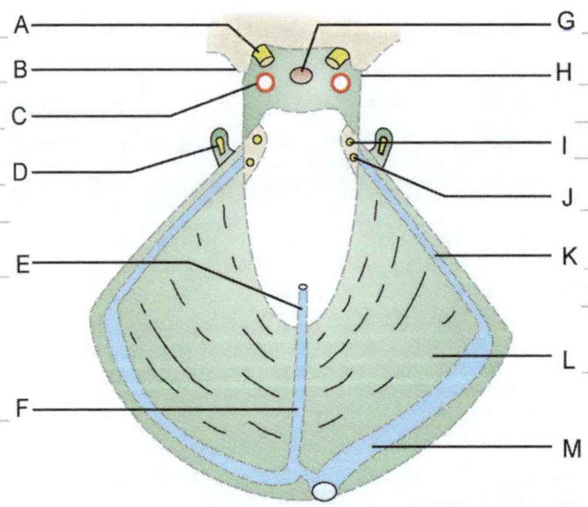


**Practice Figure 12.1:** Tentorium cerebelli and diaphragma sellae

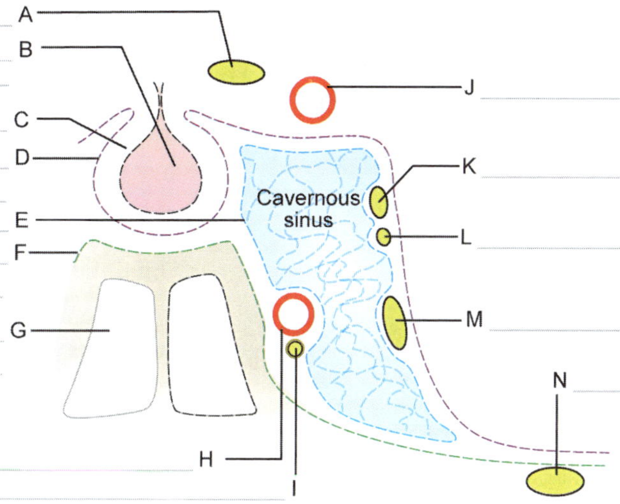


**Practice Figure 12.2:** Relations of the cavernous sinus

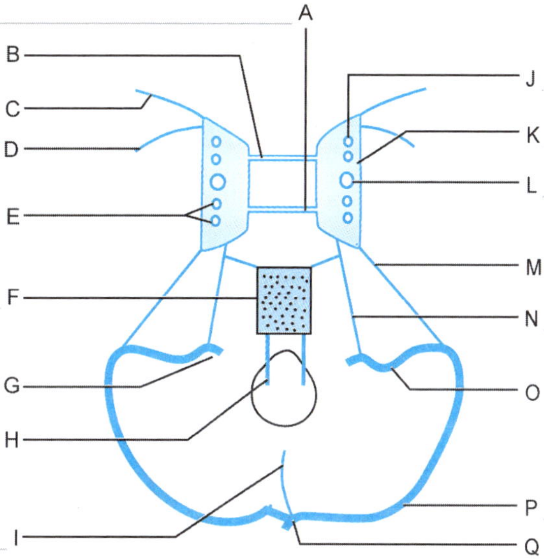


**Practice Figure 12.3:** Superior view of the tributaries and communications of the cavernous sinus

## MULTIPLE CHOICE QUESTIONS

(Tick the single best correct option)

1. Name the structure marked as X in the following image.

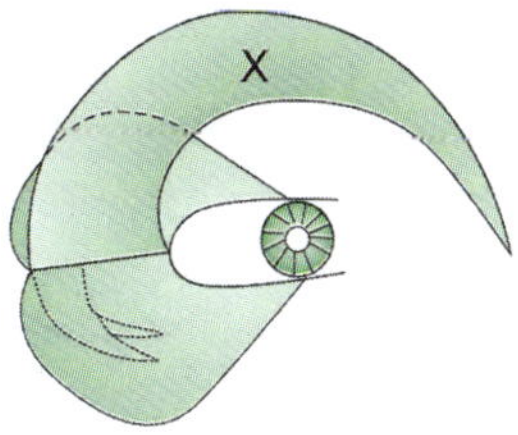


   a. Falx cerebelli
   b. Diaphragma sellae
   c. Falx cerebri
   d. Tentorium cerebelli

2. Meckel's cave contains ___________.
   a. Pterygopalatine ganglion
   b. Gasserian ganglion
   c. Celiac ganglion
   d. Superior cervical ganglion

3. Which among the following is a paired venous sinuses?
   a. Inferior petrosal sinus
   b. Superior sagittal sinus
   c. Posterior intercavernous sinus
   d. Basilar plexus of veins

4. Which nerve accompanies the internal carotid artery in the medial wall of cavernous sinus?
   a. Abducens
   b. Optic
   c. Oculomotor
   d. Mandibular

5. A 38-year-old female visited an endocrinologist with complaints of persistent headaches, tubular vision and unexplained weight gain over the past six months. Where does the tumour compresses to cause bitemporal hemianopia?
   a. Optic nerve
   b. Optic chiasma
   c. Lateral geniculate nucleus
   d. Occipital lobe

6. A 72-year-old male presented to the emergency department after experiencing a sudden episode of dizziness and loss of consciousness while turning his head to the left. After a few minutes he regained consciousness. What is the likely diagnosis?
   a. Orthostatic hypotension
   b. Carotid sinus syndrome
   c. Vasovagal syncope
   d. Cardiac arrhythmias
7. Ascending pharyngeal artery is a branch of __________.
   a. Superficial temporal artery
   b. Mandibular artery
   c. Maxillary artery
   d. External carotid artery
8. The second part of the lingual artery travels beneath __________ muscle.
   a. Geniohyoid b. Mylohyoid
   c. Hyoglossus d. Styloglossus
9. What is the significance of the carotid body?
   a. It regulates blood pressure by detecting changes in blood pressure levels
   b. It monitors blood oxygen levels and helps regulate respiratory rate
   c. It produces hormones that control heart rate
   d. It filters toxins from the blood before it reaches the brain
10. Maxillary artery and __________ are the terminal branches of the external carotid artery.
    a. Superior thyroid artery
    b. Ascending palatine artery
    c. Ascending pharyngeal artery
    d. Superficial temporal artery
11. Lesser petrosal nerve is branch of __________ nerve.
    a. Facial b. Glossopharyngeal
    c. Vagus d. Accessory
12. Injury to the middle meningeal artery may result in __________ haematoma.
    a. Subdural b. Extradural
    c. Epidural d. Subarachnoid

## QUESTION BANK

(Use separate copy to solve the following questions)

Q 1. Describe the cavernous sinus under the following headings: Boundaries, communications, tributaries, applied aspects.

Q 2. Write a short notes on:
   a. Tentorium cerebelli
   b. Superior sagittal sinus
   c. Emissary veins
   d. Blood supply of pituitary gland
   e. Middle meningeal artery
   f. Internal carotid artery
   g. Trigeminal ganglion

Q 3. Write the anatomical basis for:
   a. Pulsating exophthalmos
   b. Bitemporal hemianopia in pituitary tumours

eSmartQuiz

# Contents of the Orbit

## CLINICOANATOMICAL PROBLEMS

### Clinical Case 1

A 32-year-old female presented with sudden onset diplopia. Her right eye drifted outward and slightly downward. She reported difficulty turning her right eye inward and upward. Examination revealed ptosis and a dilated pupil on the affected side. MRI confirmed a diagnosis of **oculomotor nerve palsy**.

1. Why did the eye drift outward and slightly downward?
2. Why did the patient have difficulty turning her eye inward and upward?
3. Why did the patient have ptosis and dilated pupil?

#### Explanation

1. ____________________

2. ____________________

3. ____________________

### Clinical Case 2

A 60-year-old male experienced sudden blindness in his right eye. Ophthalmoscopic examination revealed pale retina and a cherry-red spot at the macula, indicating **occlusion of the central artery of the retina**. He also presented with papilloedema, suggesting increased intracranial pressure.

1. What has caused blindness in this particular case?
2. Name the other end arteries in the body.

#### Explanation

1. ____________________

2. ____________________

## PRACTICE FIGURES

(Label the practice figures)

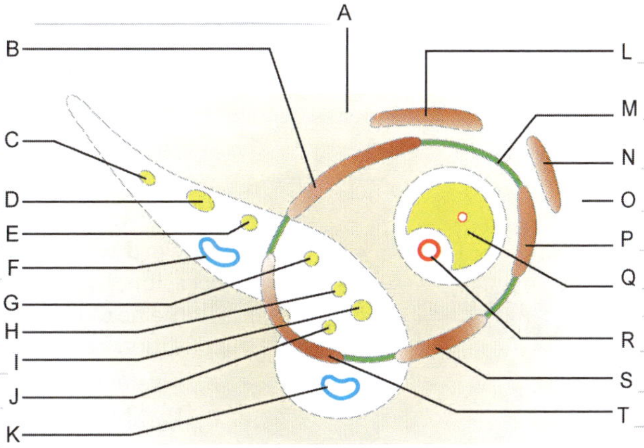


**Practice Figure 13.1:** Origin of the extraocular muscles and the structures passing through superior orbital fissure

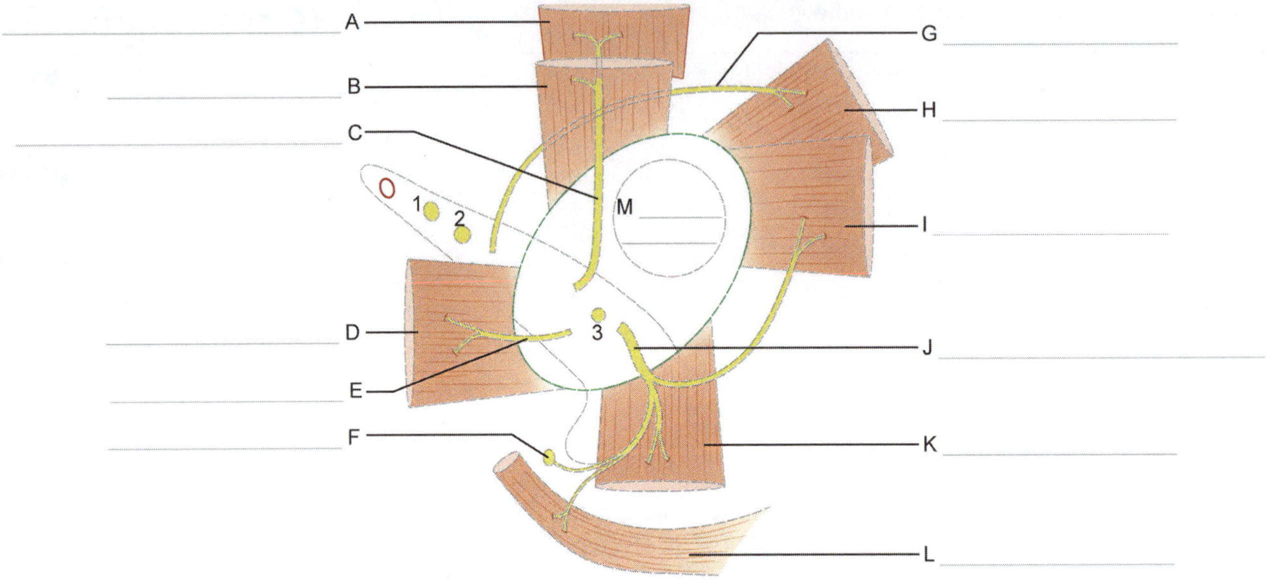


**Practice Figure 13.2:** Nerve supply of the extraocular muscles (1. Lacrimal nerve, 2. Frontal nerve, 3. Nasociliary nerve)

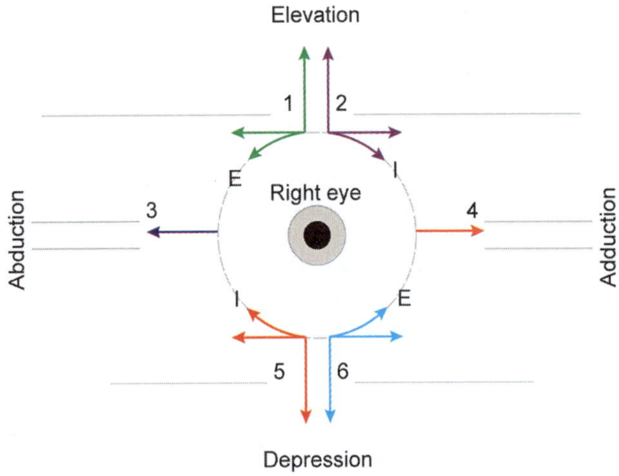


**Practice Figure 13.3:** Actions of extraocular muscles (I: Intorsion, E: Extorsion)

## MULTIPLE CHOICE QUESTIONS

(Tick the single best correct option)

1. Identify the structure marked as X.

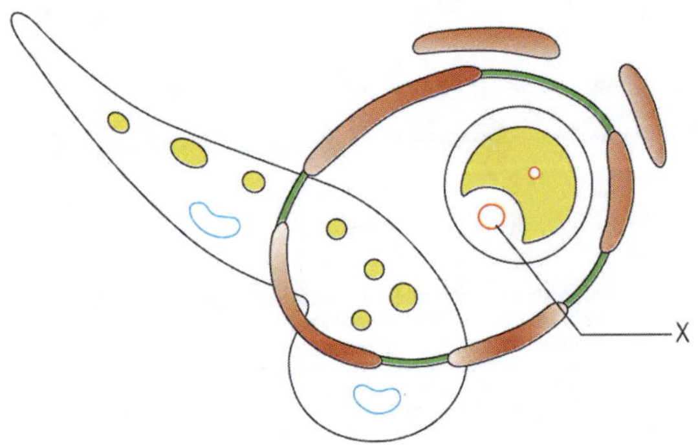


   a. Infraorbital artery
   b. Ophthalmic artery
   c. Ciliary artery
   d. Supraorbital artery

2. Suspensory ligament of Lockwood is a modification of __________.
   a. Medial check ligament
   b. Lateral check ligament
   c. Tenon's capsule
   d. Fascial sheath

3. What are the muscles responsible for the movement shown below?

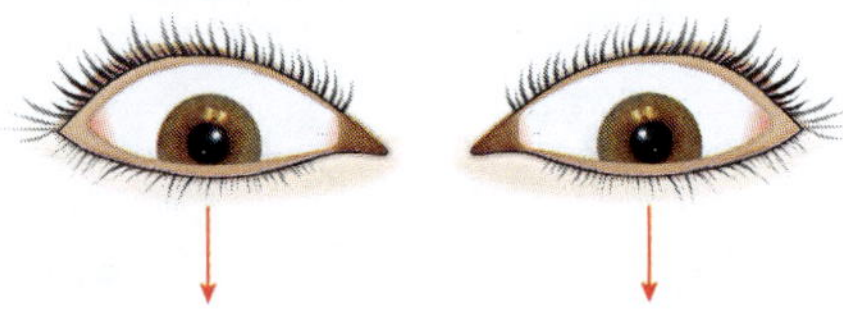

   a. Superior rectus and superior oblique
   b. Superior rectus and inferior oblique
   c. Inferior rectus and superior oblique
   d. Inferior rectus and inferior oblique

4. The posterior ethmoidal nerve is a branch of __________.
   a. Ophthalmic division of trigeminal nerve
   b. Supraorbital nerve
   c. Nasociliary nerve
   d. Supratrochlear nerve

5. What is the nerve supply of superior oblique muscle?
   a. Trochlear nerve
   b. Abducens nerve
   c. Optic nerve
   d. Oculomotor nerve

6. A 5-year-old child was brought to the clinic by their parents when they noticed that one eye seems to drift outward while the other stays focused. The child also occasionally complains of double vision and seems to tilt the head to one side to see better. What is the clinical condition known as ?
   a. Nystagmus
   b. Paralytic squint
   c. Duane retraction syndrome
   d. Concomitant squint

7. At which axis does the adduction and abduction of the cornea take place?
   a. Vertical axis
   b. Anterior-posterior axis
   c. Horizontal axis
   d. Oblique axis
8. Which cranial nerve lies in the Dorello's canal?
   a. Optic nerve
   b. Oculomotor nerve
   c. Trochlear nerve
   d. Abducens nerve
9. Following picture shows roots and branches of ciliary ganglion. Identify the structure marked as X.

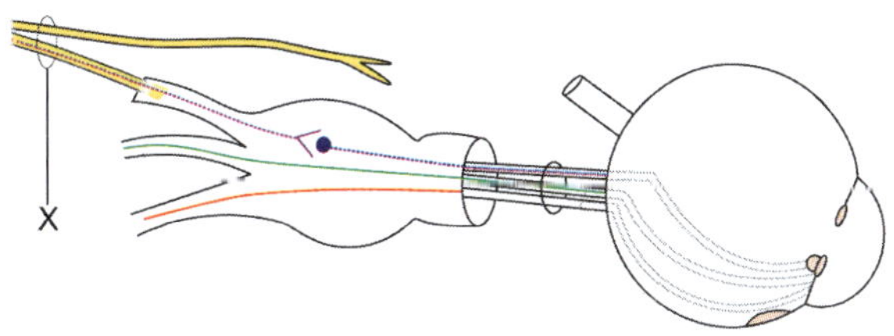


   a. Parasympathetic root
   b. Sympathetic root
   c. Nerve to inferior oblique
   d. Short ciliary nerve
10. Which of the following statements about the optic nerve is TRUE?
   a. The optic nerve is responsible for eye movement
   b. The optic nerve transmits visual information from the retina to the brain
   c. The optic nerve controls the pupil constriction reflex
   d. The optic nerve is the shortest cranial nerve

## QUESTION BANK

(Use separate copy to solve the following questions)

Q 1. Describe the extraocular muscles under the following headings: Origin, insertion, nerve supply actions, and applied aspects.

Q 2. Write a short notes on:
   a. Ciliary ganglion
   b. Ophthalmic artery
   c. Ophthalmic nerve

Chapter

14

eSmartQuiz

# Mouth and Pharynx

## CLINICOANATOMICAL PROBLEMS

### Clinical Case 1

A 11-year-old girl presented with sore throat and earache. He had 102°F temperature and difficulty in swallowing. The ENT surgeon diagnosed her as a case of **tonsillitis**.

1. Name the components of Waldeyer's lymphatic ring.
2. Explain the anatomical basis of earache in tonsillitis.
3. Name the surgery required for removal of tonsil.
4. Name the chief lymph node that drains the tonsil.

### *Explanation*

1. ______________________________

2. ______________________________

3. ______________________________

4. ______________________________

### Clinical Case 2

A 4-year-old boy was brought to the emergency room after swallowing a coin. He exhibited difficulty swallowing and mild respiratory distress. X-rays confirmed the coin lodged in the piriform fossa. An ENT specialist performed an emergency endoscopic procedure to safely remove the coin.

1. What is piriform fossa?
2. Name the nerve related to this fossa.
3. What is an alternate name for this fossa?

### *Explanation*

1. ______________________________

2. ______________________________

3. ______________________________

## PRACTICE FIGURES

(Label the practice figures)

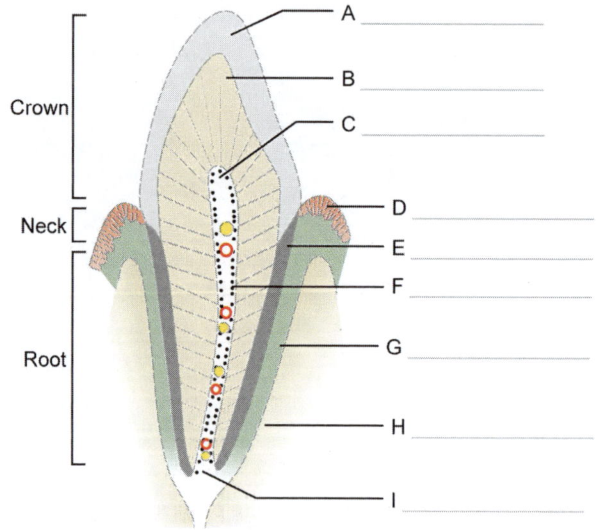


**Practice Figure 14.1:** Parts of a tooth

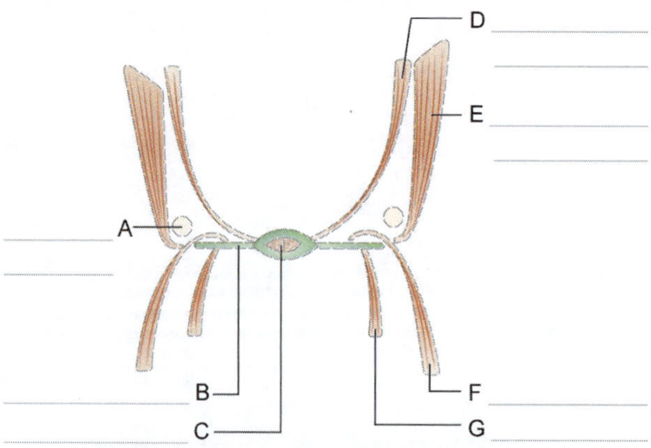


**Practice Figure 14.2:** Muscles of soft palate

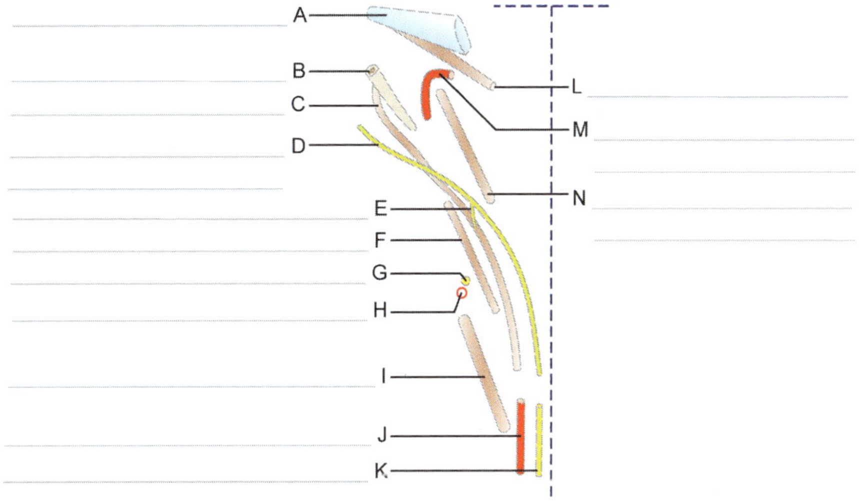


**Practice Figure 14.3:** Gaps between pharyngeal muscles and the structures related to them

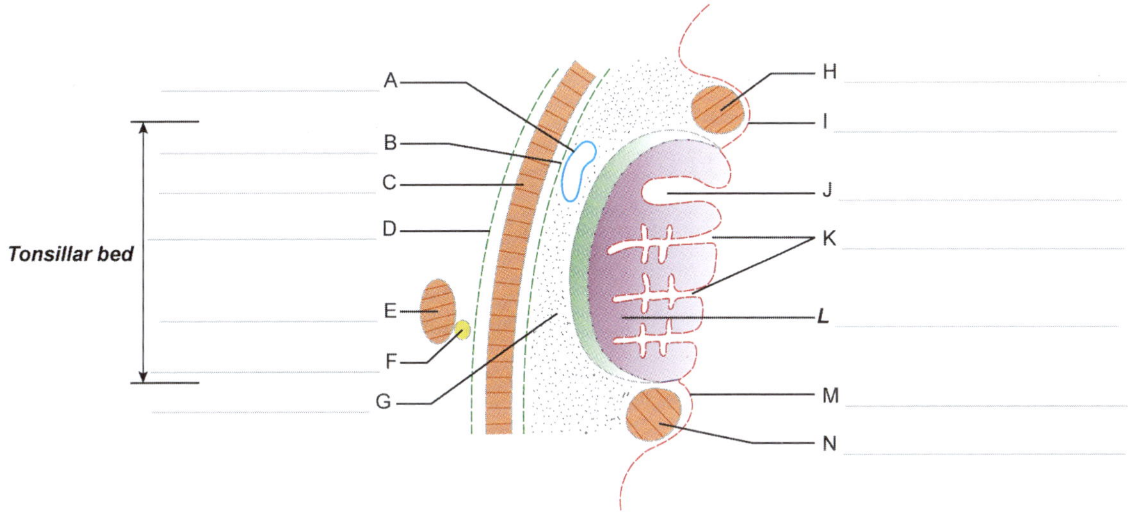


**Practice Figure 14.4:** Deep relations of tonsil

## MULTIPLE CHOICE QUESTIONS

(Tick the single best correct option)

1. The levator veli palatini muscle passes through:
   a. Gap above the superior constrictor
   b. Gap between the superior and middle constrictor
   c. Gap between the middle and inferior constrictor
   d. Gap below the inferior constrictor
2. Name the structure marked as X in the following image.

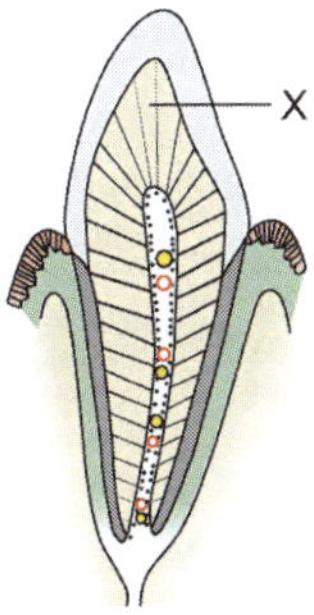


   a. Enamel b. Pulp
   c. Cement d. Dentine

3. Passavant's ridge is formed by ___________ muscle.
   a. Inferior constrictor
   b. Palatopharyngeus
   c. Stylopharyngeus
   d. Tensor veli palatini
4. Name the structure marked as X in the below image.

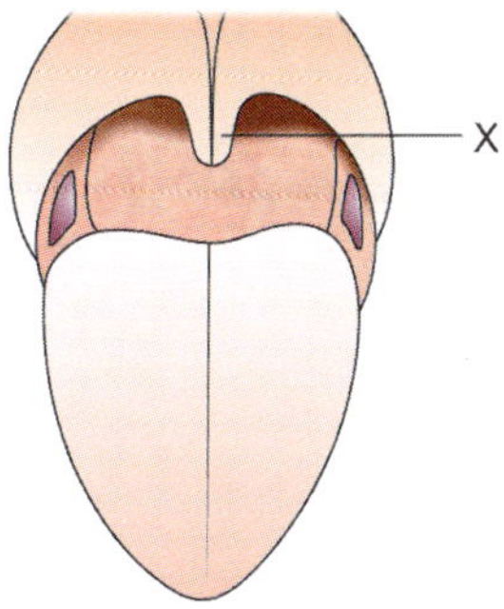


   a. Soft palate b. Uvula
   c. Palatine tonsil d. Median raphe

5. You are at a family dinner, your uncle sitting across the table, suddenly stops talking and grabs his throat. He was distressed, face was turning red, and he was unable

to cough or speak. Which of the following lifesaving procedure will you perform?
a. Cardiopulmonary resuscitation
b. Rescue breathing
c. Heimlich maneuver
d. Applying a tourniquet

6. Which among the following muscles does not belong to the soft palate?
a. Palatoglossus b. Palatopharyngeus
c. Levator palati d. Cricopharyngeus

7. Which nerve injury results in the below mentioned condition?

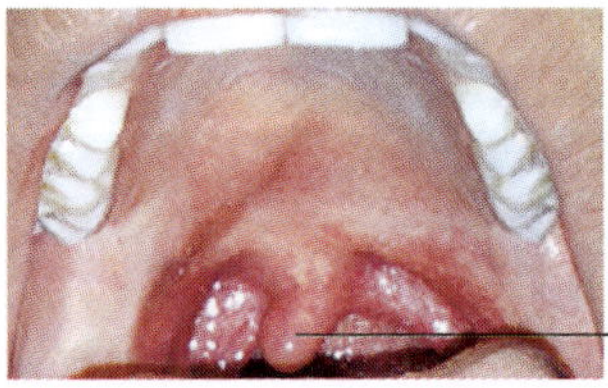


a. Right vagus
b. Left vagus
c. Right recurrent laryngeal nerve
d. Left recurrent laryngeal nerve

8. The bed of the tonsil is formed by all, EXCEPT:
a. Pharyngobasilar fascia b. Palatoglossus
c. Buccopharyngeal fascia d. Glossopharyngeal nerve

9. Pick out the CORRECT statement about the pharyngotympanic tube.
a. The bony part forms the anterior and medial two-thirds of the tube
b. The cartilaginous part forms the posterior and lateral one-third of the tube
c. Its bony part is supplied by nervus spinosus branch of the mandibular nerve
d. The tube opens during swallowing and sneezing

10. What is the nerve supply of tensor veli palatini muscle?
a. Vagus nerve b. Mandibular nerve
c. Facial nerve d. Glossopharyngeal nerve

11. Tonsillitis pain is referred to pain in ear as both are supplied by:
a. Auricular branch of vagus
b. Glossopharyngeal nerve
c. Lingual nerve
d. Accessory nerve

12. The joint between tooth and gum is:
a. Syndesmosis b. Gomphosis
c. Sutures d. Cartilaginous joint

13. All of the following structures form bed of the tonsil, EXCEPT:
a. Superior constrictor
b. Pharyngobasilar fascia
c. Buccinator muscle
d. Buccopharyngeal fascia

## QUESTION BANK

(Use separate copy to solve the following questions)

Q 1. Describe the muscles of soft palate under the following headings: Origin, insertion, nerve supply, actions, and applied aspects.

Q 2. Describe the constrictor muscles of pharynx under the following headings: Origin, insertion, nerve supply, actions, and applied aspects.

Q 3. Describe the palatine tonsil under the following headings: Gross features, bed of tonsil, blood supply, nerve supply, and applied aspects.

Q 4. Write a short notes on:
a. Waldeyer's ring
b. Auditory tube
c. Muscles of soft palate
d. Piriform fossa
e. Foramen of Morgagni
f. Pharyngeal plexus
g. Buccopharyngeal membrane
h. Cleft palate
i. Killian dehiscence.

Chapter

15

# Nose, Paranasal Sinuses and Pterygopalatine Fossa

eSmartQuiz

## CLINICOANATOMICAL PROBLEM

### Clinical Case 1

A 10-year-old boy experienced sudden nosebleeds during a heatwave. He was playing outside when his nose started bleeding profusely. His parents managed to stop the bleeding temporarily and brought him to the clinic. The doctor diagnosed him with **epistaxis**.

1. What is the location of Kiesselbach's plexus?
2. Name the arteries forming Kiesselbach's plexus.
3. Which artery is called artery of nose bleeding?

*Explanation*

1. ______________________________

2. ______________________________

3. ______________________________

## PRACTICE FIGURES

(Label the practice figures)

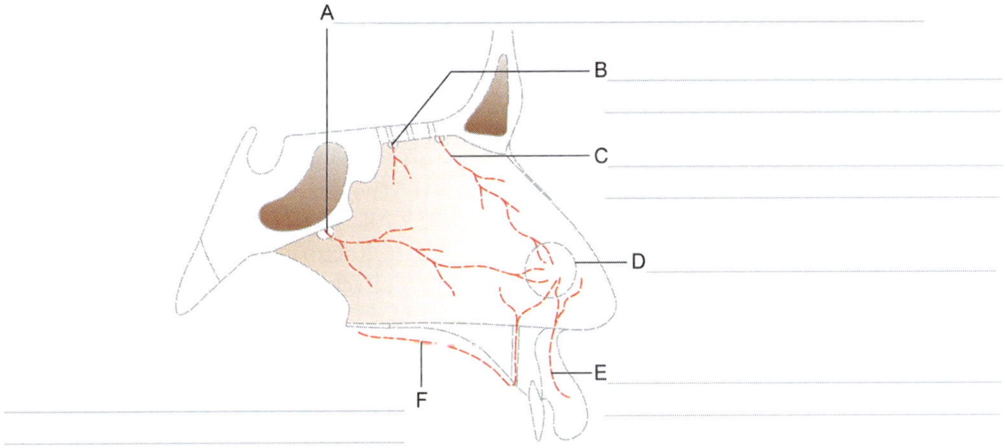


**Practice Figure 15.1:** Arterial supply of nasal septum

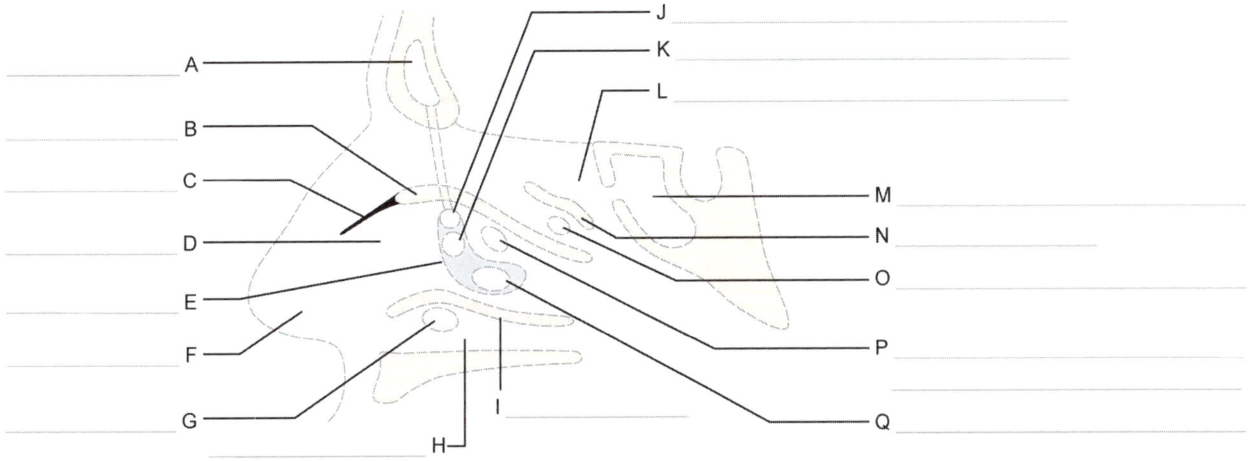


**Practice Figure 15.2:** Lateral wall of the nasal cavity seen after removing the conchae

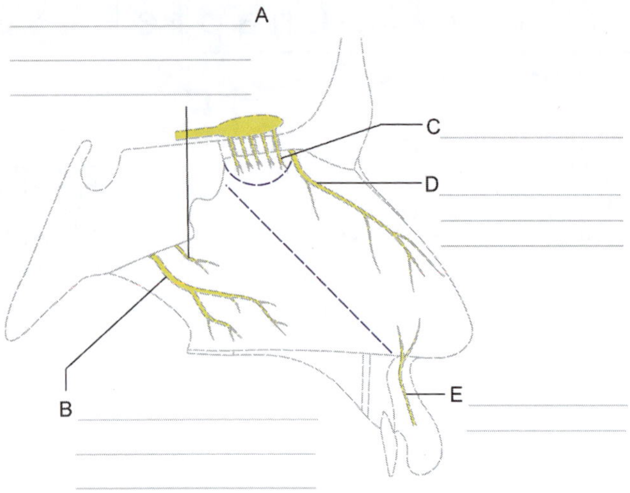


**Practice Figure 15.3:** Nerve supply of the nasal septum

## MULTIPLE CHOICE QUESTIONS

(Tick the single best correct option)

1. Nasal septum is formed by all of the following structures, EXCEPT?
   a. Vomer
   b. Perpendicular plate of ethmoid
   c. Septal cartilage
   d. Maxillary bone
2. Vidian's nerve is ___________.
   a. Greater petrosal nerve + zygomaticotemporal nerve
   b. Deep petrosal nerve + lacrimal nerve
   c. Zygomaticotemporal nerve + lacrimal nerve
   d. Greater petrosal nerve + deep petrosal nerve
3. Identify the clinical condition shown below.

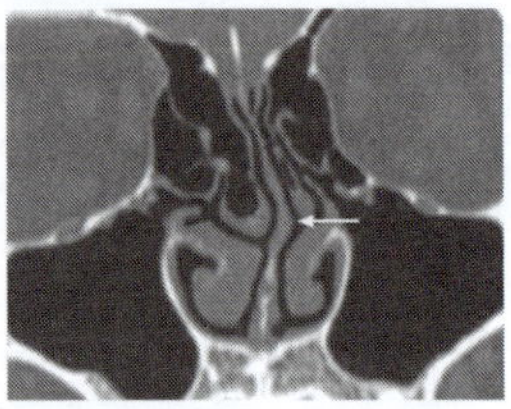

   a. Septal haemorrhage
   b. Deviated nasal septum
   c. Septal perforation
   d. Carcinoma of nasal cavity
4. Which is the largest of all the paranasal sinuses?
   a. Frontal sinus
   b. Ethmoidal sinus
   c. Maxillary sinus
   d. Sphenoidal sinus
5. Which of the following is not a content of pterygopalatine fossa?
   a. Maxillary nerve
   b. 3rd part of maxillary artery
   c. Pterygopalatine ganglion
   d. Infraorbital nerve.
6. A 30-year-old male met with an accident one month back. He has complaints of clear, watery nasal discharge, primarily from the left nostril. Which increases with physical activity or bending forwards. What is the most likely diagnosis?
   a. CSF rhinorrhoea
   b. Sinusitis
   c. Allergic rhinitis
   d. Nasal polyps
7. Identify the structure marked as X.

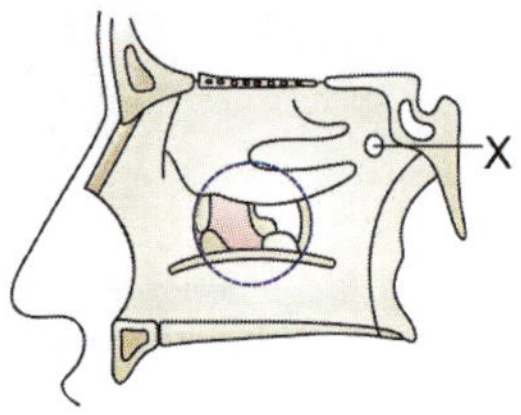


   a. Frontal process of maxilla
   b. Uncinate process of ethmoid
   c. Sphenopalatine foramen
   d. Medial pterygoid plate
8. Which of the following structures is not a component of the osteomeatal complex?
   a. Uncinate process
   b. Middle turbinate
   c. Ethmoid bulla
   d. Sphenoid sinus
9. Anteroinferior quadrant of the lateral nasal wall is supplied by ___________.
   a. Anterior superior alveolar nerve
   b. Anterior ethmoidal nerve
   c. Posterior ethmoidal nerve
   d. Anterior palatine nerve
10. Which of the following statements about olfactory nerves is true?
    a. Olfactory cells are unipolar neurons.
    b. The olfactory nerves are about 30 in number.
    c. Allergic rhinitis causes permanent olfactory impairment.
    d. Olfactory nerves transmit signals directly to the olfactory cortex in the brain.
11. ___________ sinus is the first air sinus to develop.
    a. Maxillary
    b. Ethmoidal
    c. Frontal
    d. Sphenoidal

## QUESTION BANK

(Use separate copy to solve the following questions)

Q 1. Discuss the features of lateral wall of nose.

Q 2. Write a short notes on:
   a. Maxillary air sinus into nasal cavity
   b. Maxillary nerve
   c. Pterygopalatine ganglion
   d. The most common site of bleed on medial wall of nose
   e. Pterygopalatine ganglion

Q 3. Draw a well labelled diagram showing
   a. Blood supply and nerve supply of the medial wall of nose
   b. Blood supply and nerve supply of the lateral wall of nose
   c. Openings of paranasal air sinuses in the lateral wall of nose.

eSmartQuiz

# Larynx

## CLINICOANATOMICAL PROBLEM

### Clinical Case 1

A 5-year-old boy accidentally inhaled a small toy at a birthday party. He became unable to breathe and started turning blue. A physician at the party immediately examined and quickly performed the Heimlich manoeuvre, successfully dislodging the toy from the larynx.

1. Why did a boy have difficulty in breathing?
2. What is Heimlich manoeuvre?
3. Which is the narrowest part of the larynx?

### *Explanation*

1. ____________________

2. ____________________

3. ____________________

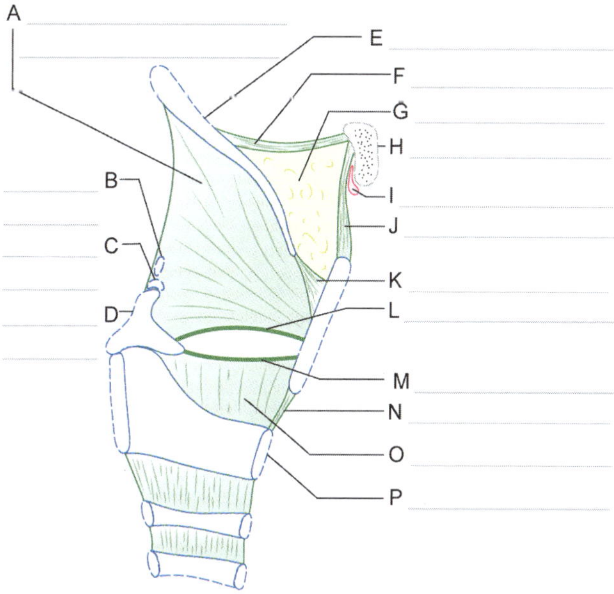


**Practice Figure 16.2:** Ligaments and membranes of larynx

## PRACTICE FIGURES

(Label the practice figures)

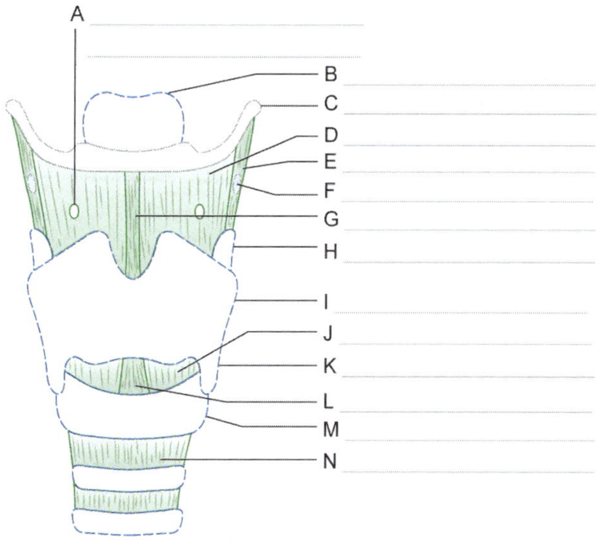


**Practice Figure 16.1:** Cartilages and skeleton of larynx

## MULTIPLE CHOICE QUESTIONS

(Tick the single best correct option)

1. How much cartilage does the larynx contain?
   a. 8 b. 7
   c. 9 d. 6

2. Depression of larynx is caused by __________.
   a. Sternothyroid
   b. Cricothyroid
   c. Thyrohyoid
   d. Aryepiglottic

3. Who is prone to develop the below mentioned clinical condition?

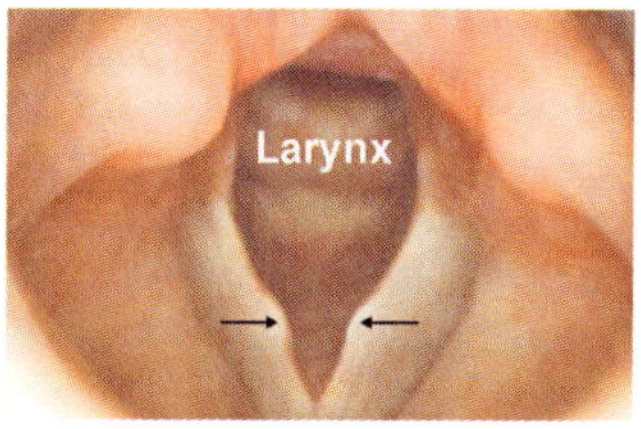


   a. Gastroesophageal reflux disease
   b. Singers
   c. Infants
   d. People with asthma

4. What is the action of the muscle marked with X?

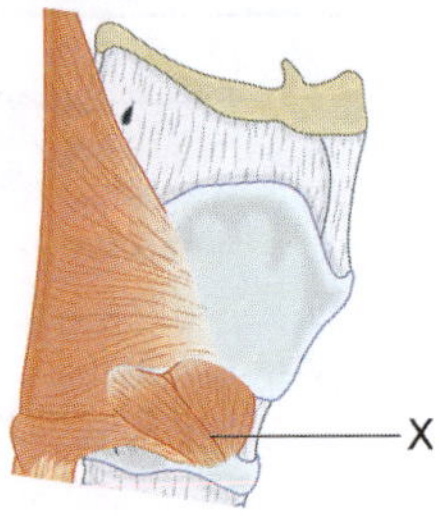


a. Tensor of vocal cord b. Adductor of vocal cord
c. Abductor of vocal cord d. Relaxor of vocal cord

5. Name the structure marked by X.

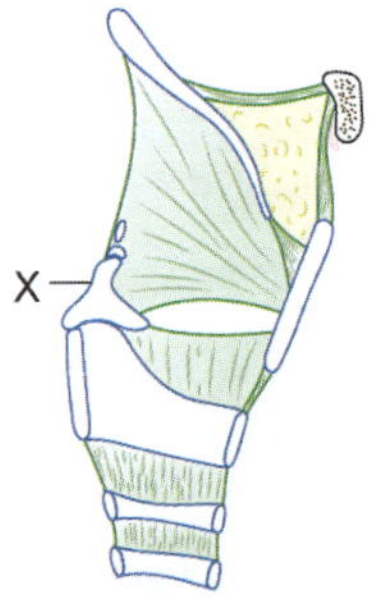


a. Arytenoid cartilage b. Cricothyroid joint
c. Thyroid cartilage d. Epiglottis

6. __________ is the only abductor of the vocal cord.
   a. Lateral cricoarytenoid
   b. Thyroarytenoid
   c. Posterior cricoarytenoid
   d. Cricothyroid

7. Identify the nerve marked as X.

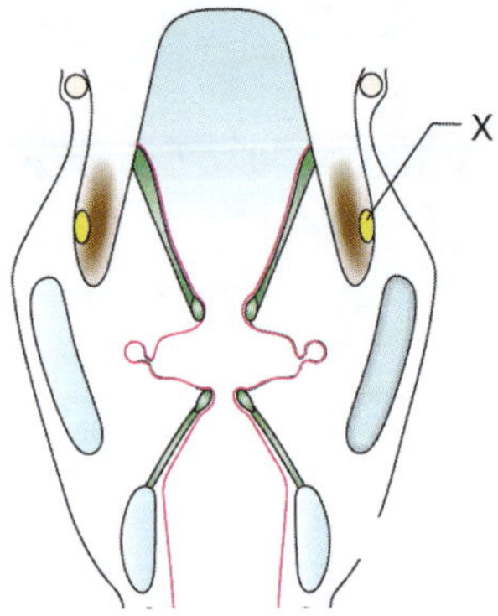


a. Recurrent laryngeal nerve
b. External laryngeal nerve
c. Internal laryngeal nerve
d. Vagus nerve

8. A 50-year-old male was admitted in the emergency department with a history of loss of consciousness for two hours following a head injury. On examination, his airway was patent, but his Glasgow Coma Scale (GCS) score was 3/12. Endotracheal intubation was planned for the patient. Where should the tube be inserted?
   a. Above the vocal cords
   b. Between the vocal cords
   c. Below the vocal cords
   d. Beside the vocal cords

9. Which membrane is pierced during a laryngotomy?
   a. Thyrohyoid membrane
   b. Cricothyroid membrane
   c. Quadrangular membrane
   d. Conus elasticus

10. What will be the position of the vocal cords if both recurrent laryngeal nerves are interrupted?
    a. Fully abducted
    b. Fully adducted
    c. Cadaveric position
    d. Median position

11. The lower margin of __________ forms the vestibular ligament of the larynx.
    a. Median thyrohyoid ligament
    b. Lateral thyrohyoid ligament
    c. Cricothyroid ligament
    d. Quadrangular membrane

12. __________ nerve supplies the mucous membrane of the larynx below the vocal folds.
    a. Pharyngeal
    b. Recurrent laryngeal
    c. Internal laryngeal
    d. External laryngeal

## QUESTION BANK

(Use separate copy to solve the following questions)

Q 1. Write a short notes on:
   a. Actions of muscle of larynx
   b. Interior of larynx
   c. Rima glottidis
   d. Conus elasticus
   e. Piriform fossa
   f. Thyroid cartilage
   g. Vocal cords

Q 2. Write the anatomical basis for:
   a. Posterior cricoarytenoid is the safety muscle of the larynx
   b. Singer's nodule

eSmartQuiz

# Tongue

## CLINICOANATOMICAL PROBLEM

### Clinical Case 1

A 45-year-old patient undergone a surgery for treatment of a middle ear infection. Following the procedure, the patient reported altered taste sensation on the front two-thirds of the tongue, accompanied by mild dryness in the mouth. The physician diagnosed him as a case of an isolated injury to the chorda tympani nerve.

1. From which nerve does the chorda tympani branch originate?
2. Why did the patient experience
   a. A altered of taste sensation in the anterior two-thirds of the tongue?
   b. Mild dryness of mouth?

*Explanation*

1. ______
2. a. ______
   b. ______

## PRACTICE FIGURES

(Label the practice figures)

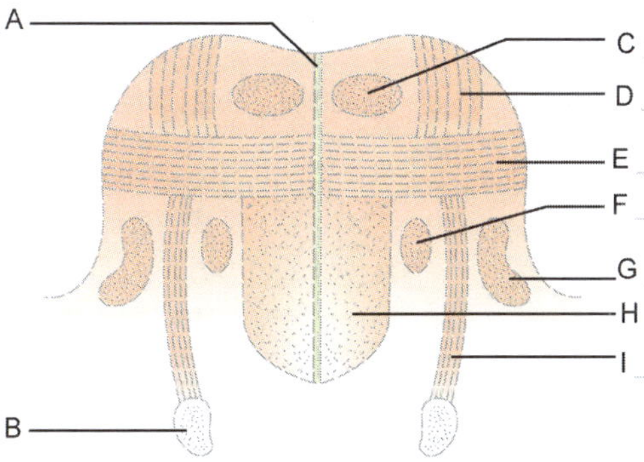


**Practice Figure 17.1:** Intrinsic and extrinsic muscles of tongue

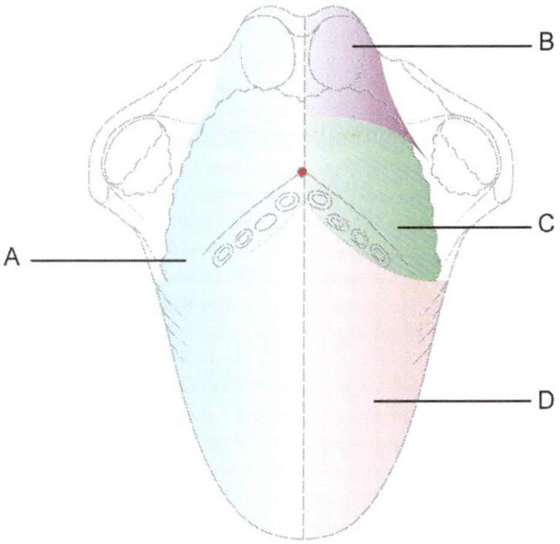


**Practice Figure 17.2:** Nerve supply of tongue

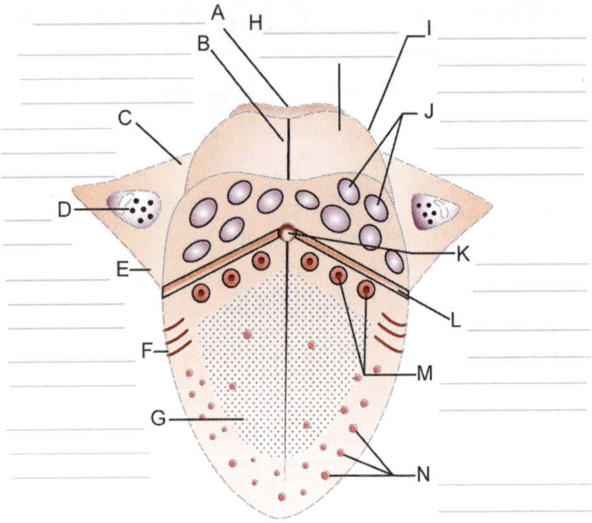


**Practice Figure 17.3:** Dorsum of the tongue, epiglottis and palatine tonsil

## MULTIPLE CHOICE QUESTIONS

(Tick the single best correct option)

1. The structure marked as X is the remnant of ________.

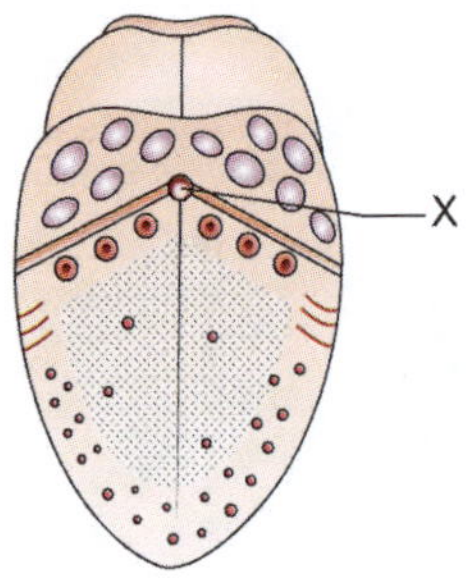


   a. Embryonic thyroid diverticulum
   b. Persistent ductus arteriosus
   c. Foramen ovale
   d. Thyroglossal duct

2. ________ is the main lymphatic drainage of the tongue.
   a. Jugulo-digastric  b. Jugulo-omohyoid
   c. Preauricular  d. Parotid lymph node

3. Palatoglossus is supplied by which nerve ________.
   a. Cranial root of accessory nerve
   b. Lingual nerve
   c. Hypoglossal nerve
   d. Vagus nerve

4. The nerve of general sensation and taste for the posterior one-third of tongue including circumvallate papillae is carried by ________.
   a. Chorda tympani nerve
   b. Glossopharyngeal nerve
   c. Vagus nerve
   d. Hypoglossal nerve

5. A 56-year-old male rushed to the emergency department with a history of chest pain, palpitation, sweating for the past 15 minutes. He was diagnosed with a myocardial infarction. Which route is preferred to administer the drug in the above mentioned situation?
   a. Sublingual  b. Intramuscular
   c. Intravenous  d. Per rectum

6. Identify the muscle marked as X.

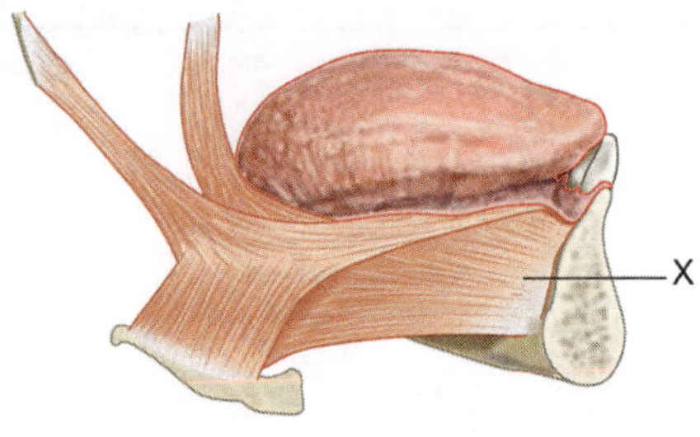


   a. Hyoglossus  b. Genioglossus
   c. Palatoglossus  d. Styloglossus

7. Which of the following is related to the taste pathway?
   a. Nucleus ambiguus  b. Nucleus solitarius
   c. Nucleus gracilis  d. Nucleus cuneatus

8. What happens to the position of the tongue when the right hypoglossal nerve gets damaged?
   a. Tongue deviates to the left
   b. Tongue remains in the midline
   c. Tongue deviates to the right
   d. Tongue shows signs of atrophy on the right side

9. Identify the true statement regarding papillae of the tongue.
   a. Circumvallate papillae are situated behind the sulcus terminalis
   b. Taste buds are numerous over the foliate papillae and over the posterior one-third of the tongue
   c. Fungiform papillae are numerous in the posterior one-third of the tongue
   d. Filiform papillae are the largest among all the papillae

10. Which of the following is not the intrinsic muscles of the tongue?
    a. Palatoglossus
    b. Superior longitudinal
    c. Hyoglossus
    d. Genioglossus

11. The muscle which protrudes the tongue and its tip toward the opposite side is:
    a. Hyoglossus  b. Genioglossus
    c. Palatoglossus  d. Styloglossus

12. The nerve which carries sensations of taste from the area of the tongue posterior to the row of vallate papillae is:
    a. Chorda tympani nerve
    b. Vagus nerve
    c. Glossopharyngeal nerve
    d. Hypoglossal nerve

## QUESTION BANK

(Use separate copy to solve the following questions)

Q 1. Describe the tongue under the following headings: gross features, muscles of tongue, nerve supply, blood supply and applied aspects.

Q 2. Write a short notes on:
   a. Nerve supply of tongue
   b. Lymphatic drainage of tongue

Q 3. Write the anatomical basis for:
   a. Hypoglossal nerve palsy
   b. Circumvallate papillae are supplied by glossopharyngeal nerve
   c. Genioglossus is a safety muscle of tongue

eSmartQuiz

# Ear

## CLINICOANATOMICAL PROBLEM

### Clinical Case 1

A 7-year-old girl was brought to the doctor with complaints of a sore throat, fever and bilateral earache. On examination, her tonsils were found to be enlarged and inflamed. An otoscopy revealed congested and reddish eardrums, particularly on the right side. The physician diagnosed her with acute otitis media and pharyngotonsillitis.

1. What is otitis media?
2. How does an infection from tonsillitis spread to the middle ear cavity?
3. What are the normal findings observed during an otoscopy?

### Explanation

1. ____________________

2. ____________________

3. ____________________

## PRACTICE FIGURES

(Label the practice figures)

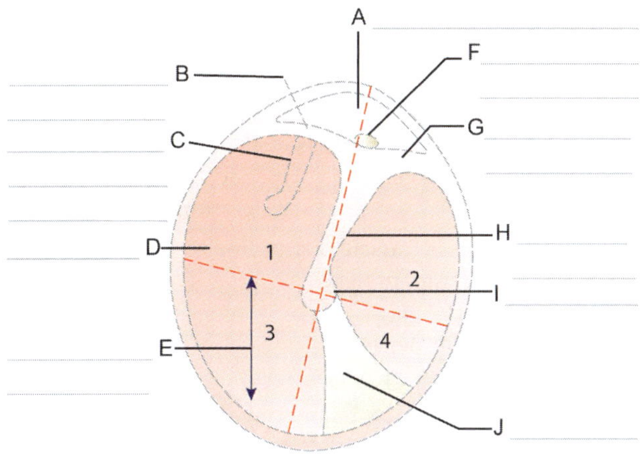


**Practice Figure 18.1:** Tympanic membrane (1) Posterosuperior quadrant; (2) Anterosuperior quadrant; (3) Posteroinferior quadrant; (4) Anteroinferior quadrant

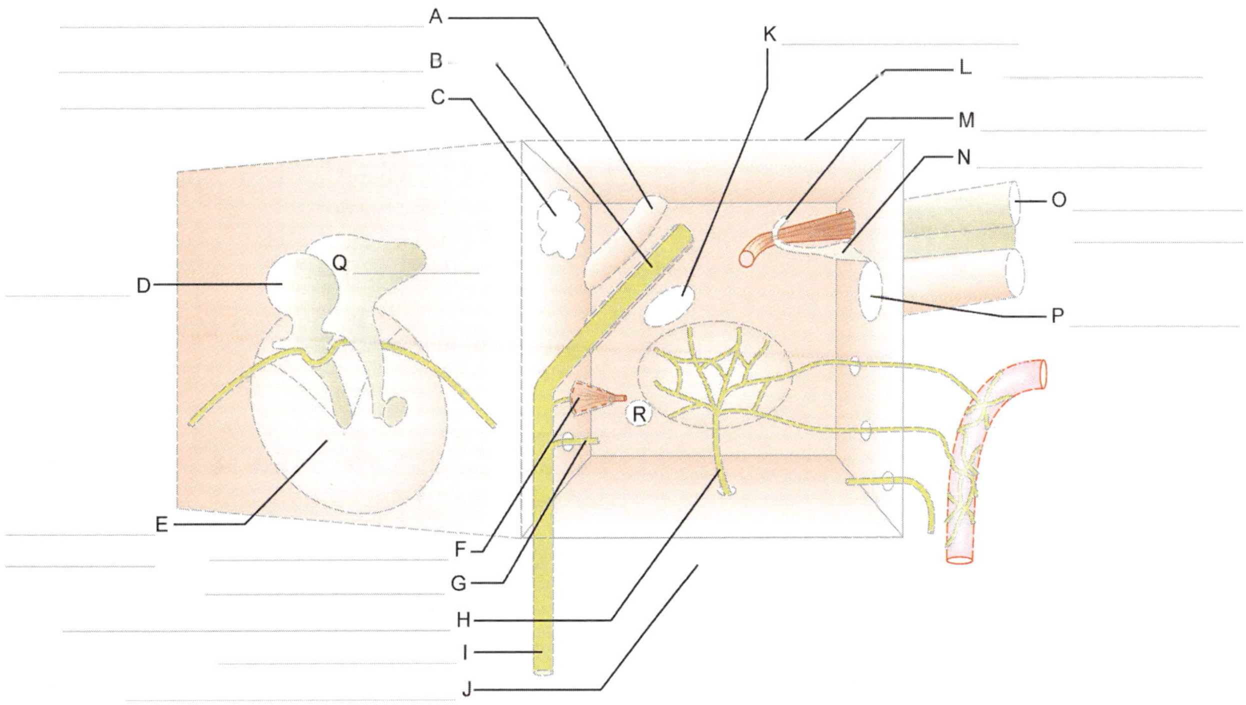


**Practice Figure 18.2:** Walls of middle ear (right middle ear, R: round window)

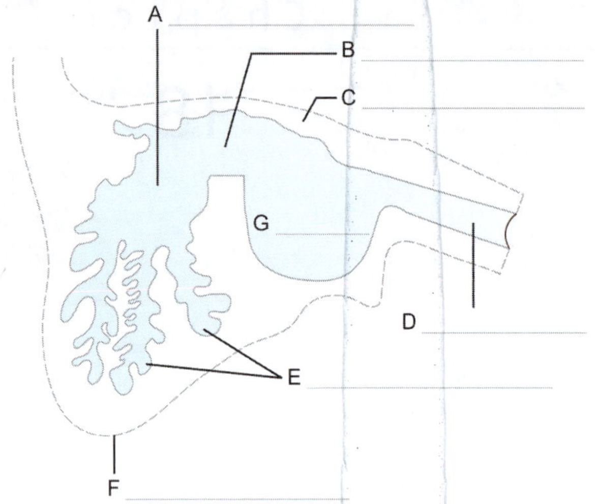


**Practice Figure 18.3:** Mastoid antrum and mastoid air cells

## MULTIPLE CHOICE QUESTIONS

(Tick the single best correct option)

1. The incudostapedial joint is a ____________ joint.
   a. Ball and socket  b. Saddle
   c. Hinge  d. Gliding
2. Tensor tympani muscle is supplied by ____________.
   a. Chorda tympani nerve
   b. Facial nerve
   c. Mandibular nerve
   d. Spinal accessory nerve
3. The structure shown below develops from ____________.

   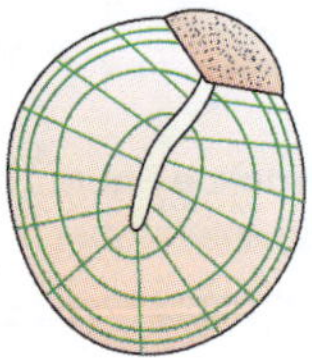

   a. Endoderm
   b. Ectoderm
   c. Mesoderm
   d. All of the above
4. The floor of the middle ear cavity is formed by:

   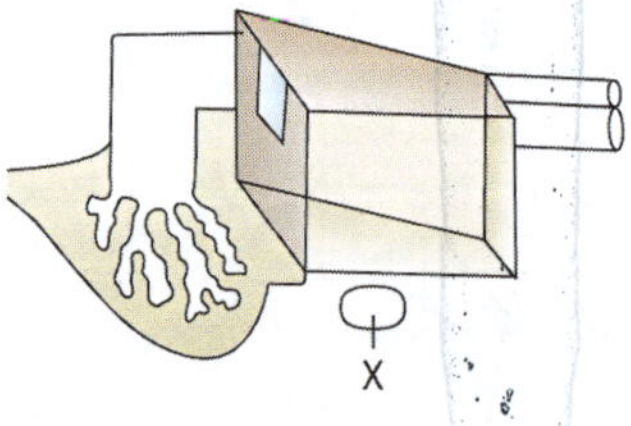
   

   a. Jugular bulb
   b. Internal carotid artery
   c. Canal for facial nerve
   d. Chorda tympani nerve
5. Identify the structure marked as X.

   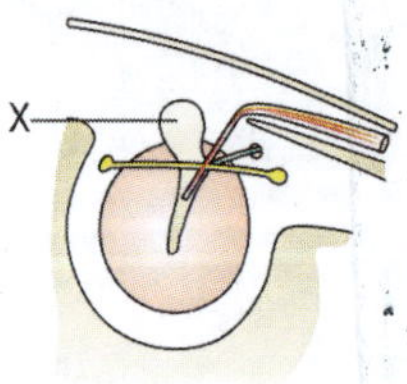
   

   a. Incus  b. Stapes
   c. Stapedius  d. Malleus
6. All of the following are features of the medial wall of the middle ear, EXCEPT:
   a. Fenestra vestibule  b. Promontory
   c. Sinus tympani  d. Petrotympanic fissure
7. A 45-year-old male patient presented to the outpatient clinic with complaints of a sensation of fullness and decreased hearing in his left ear for the past week. On examination, the otolaryngologist finds a large amount of ear wax completely occluding the external auditory canal. During syringing procedure, the patient suddenly complains of dizziness and lightheadedness. What is the most likely cause ?
   a. Middle ear infection
   b. Perforation of the tympanic membrane
   c. Vasovagal response
   d. Sudden drop in blood pressure due to dehydration
8. Which of the following statements about the semicircular canal is true?
   a. The semicircular canals are filled with air to detect changes in head position
   b. Each semicircular canal detects rotational movements in one of three planes
   c. The semicircular canals are located in the middle ear and are part of the auditory system
   d. The semicircular canals have no role in maintaining balance and equilibrium
9. Identify the space marked as X.

   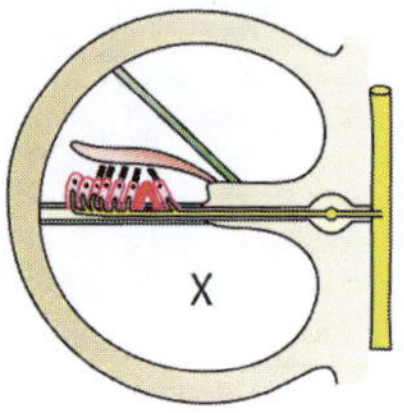
   

   a. Scala vestibuli  b. Scala tympani
   c. Tunnel of Corti  d. Space for spiral ganglion
10. Endolymph is produced by ____________.
    a. Organ of Corti  b. Reissner's membrane
    c. Stria vascularis  d. Tectorial membrane
11. The pyramid of the middle ear:
    a. Encloses the stapedius muscle.
    b. Indicates where the chorda tympani nerve enters the tympanic cavity.
    c. Is formed by the basal turn of the cochlea.
    d. Is on the medial wall of the tympanic cavity.
12. Which of the following nerve supplies stapedius muscle?
    a. Oculomotor  b. Trochlear
    c. Trigeminal  d. Facial

## QUESTION BANK

(Use separate copy to solve the following questions)

Q 1. Describe the middle ear under the following headings: Walls, content and communications.

Q 2. Write a short notes on:
   a. Mastoid antrum
   b. Otitis media
   c. Tympanic membrane
   d. Chochlea

Chapter

19

# Eyeball

eSmartQuiz

## CLINICOANATOMICAL PROBLEM

### Clinical Case 1

A 60-year-old man experienced sudden flashes of light and a shadow descending over his vision. He visited the ophthalmologist, who performed a detailed examination and diagnosed him with **retinal detachment**. The specialist explained that the retina had separated from its underlying tissue, requiring urgent surgical intervention to prevent permanent vision loss.

1. What is retinal detachment?
2. Name the main artery that supply the retina.
3. What is the optic disc in retina?

*Explanation*

1. ______

2. ______

3. ______

## PRACTICE FIGURES

(Label the practice figures)

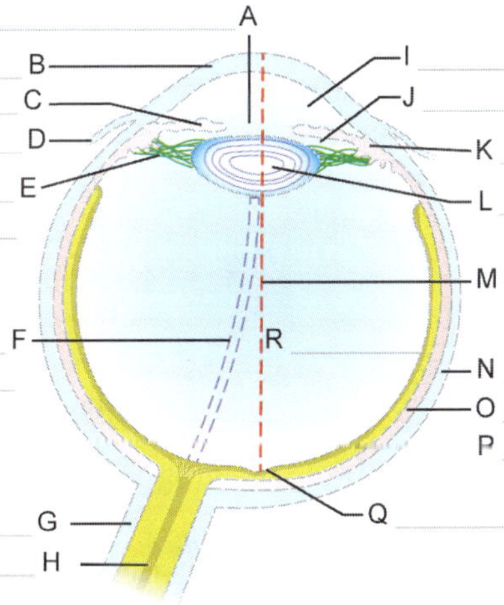


**Practice Figure 19.1:** Sagittal section of the eyeball

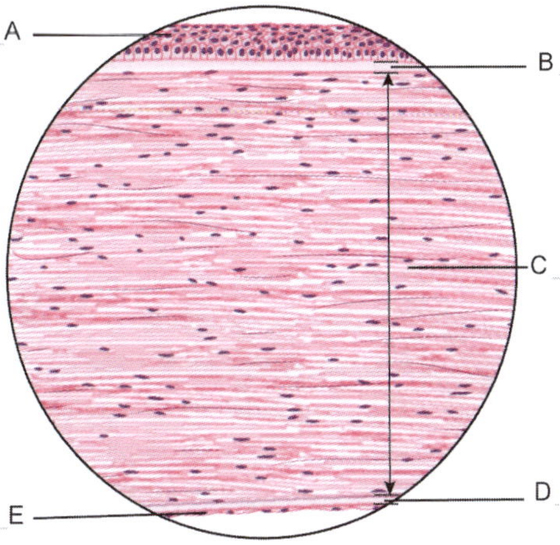


**Practice Figure 19.2:** Histology of cornea

## MULTIPLE CHOICE QUESTIONS

(Tick the single best correct option)

1. Where is the aqueous humour secreted from?
   a. Lacrimal glands
   b. Canal of Schlemm
   c. Ciliary processes
   d. Anterior ciliary veins
2. Identify the structure marked as X.

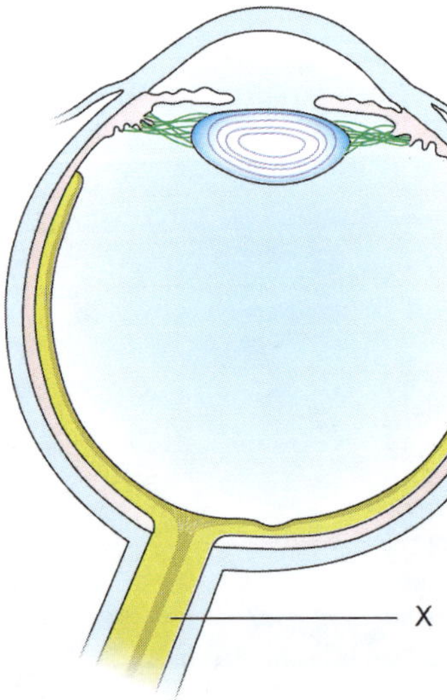


   a. Optic disc  b. Optic tract
   c. Optic nerve  d. Retina
3. A 70-year-old male patient presented to the ophthalmology clinic with complaints of progressive vision loss in both eyes over the past one year. Upon examination, the ophthalmologist observes that both lenses are opaque. What is the likely cause ?
   a. Glaucoma
   b. Macular degeneration
   c. Cataract
   d. Retinitis pigmentosa
4. Where does the choroid merge with the ciliary body?
   a. At the optic nerve
   b. At the ora serrata
   c. At the suprachoroidal lamina
   d. At the vascular lamina
5. Which artery pierce the sclera near the limbus?
   a. Posterior ciliary artery
   b. Anterior ciliary artery
   c. Venae vorticosae
   d. Muscular artery
6. What is the name of the sieve-like region at the entrance of the optic nerve?
   a. Tenon's capsule
   b. Lamina fusca
   c. Lamina cribrosa
   d. Perichoroidal space
7. What happens to the ciliary muscle and lens while looking at an object in the distance?
   a. Ciliary muscle contracts, lens becomes more convex
   b. Ciliary muscle relaxes, lens becomes flat
   c. Ciliary muscle contracts, lens becomes flat
   d. Ciliary muscle relaxes, lens becomes more convex
8. Which nerve supplies the ciliary muscle?
   a. Long ciliary nerve  b. Optic nerve
   c. Short ciliary nerve  d. Oculomotor nerve
9. From the image shown, below identify the condition.

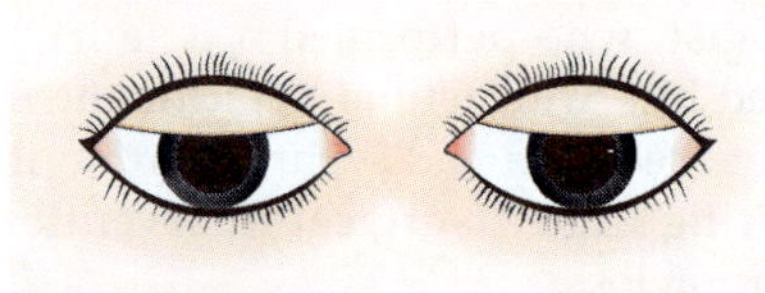

   a. Third nerve paralysis  b. Horner's syndrome
   c. Brain stem death  d. Hyperthyroidism
10. Which layer of the retina contains the photoreceptor cells responsible for detecting light?
    a. Outer nuclear layer
    b. Ganglion cell layer
    c. Inner nuclear layer
    d. Layer of rods and cones
11. Which of the following nerves supplies the cornea?
    a. Supraorbital
    b. Nasociliary
    c. Lacrimal
    d. Infraorbital
12. One of the following symptoms is not seen in Horner's syndrome:
    a. Partial ptosis
    b. Miosis
    c. Anhydrosis
    d. Exophthalmos

## QUESTION BANK

(Use separate copy to solve the following question)

Q 1. Write a short notes on:
   a. Cornea
   b. Layers of retina
   c. Lens
   d. Sclerochorneal junction

# Surface Marking and Radiological Anatomy

eSmartQuiz

## PRACTICE FIGURES

(Label the practice figures)

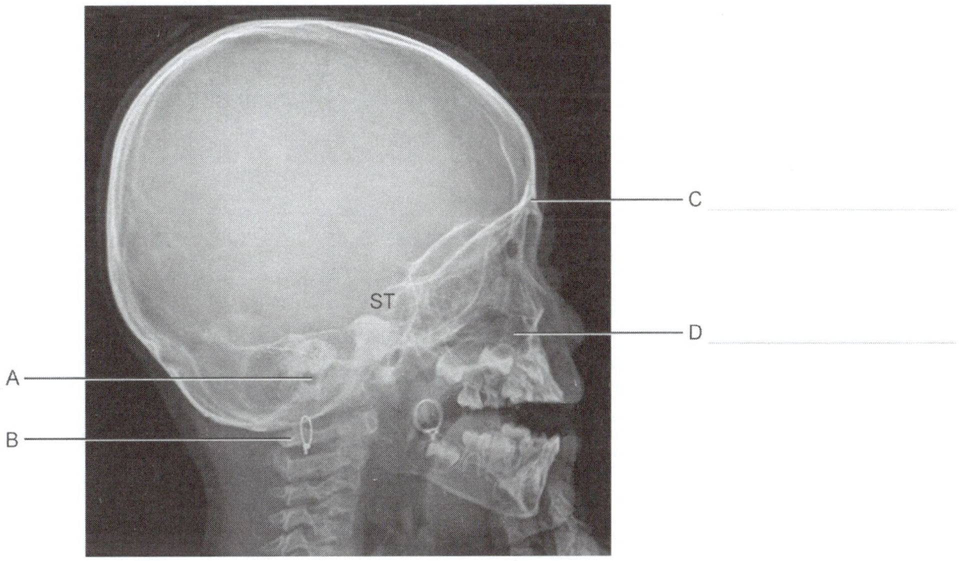


**Practice Figure 20.1:** Plane radiograph of skull: Lateral view

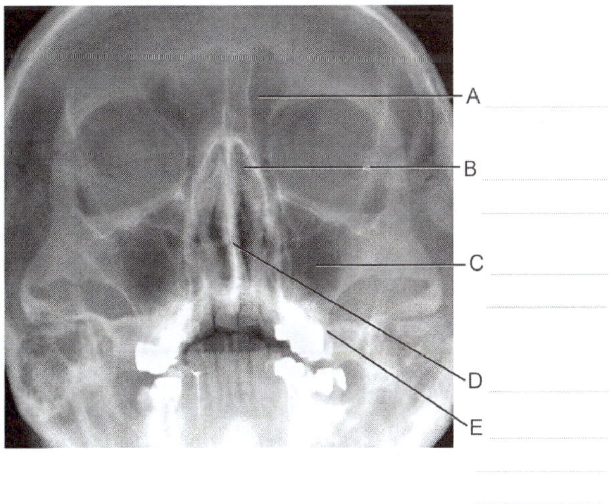


**Practice Figure 20.2:** X-ray of skull showing paranasal sinuses (Water's view/occipitomental view)

## MULTIPLE CHOICE QUESTIONS

(Tick the single best correct option)

1. Identify the structure marked as X in the picture.

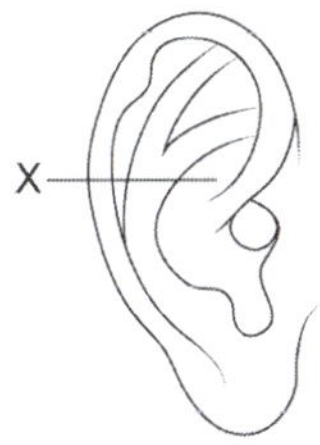


   a. Tragus
   b. Triangular fossa
   c. Cymba conchae
   d. Darwin's tubercle

2. What does Frankfurt's plane represent?
   a. The anterior end of the upper border of the zygomatic arch
   b. A slight depression in the lateral orbital margin
   c. A curved line extending from the head of the mandible to the anterior end of the zygomatic arch
   d. A horizontal line from the infraorbital margin to the external acoustic meatus

3. Name the structure marked by X.

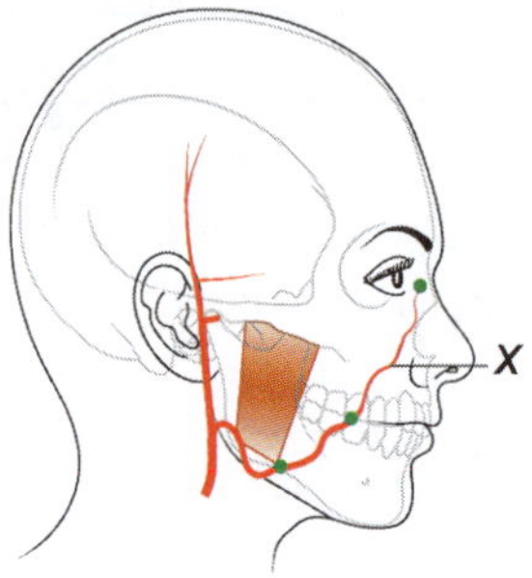


a. External carotid artery b. Lingual artery
c. Maxillary artery d. Facial artery

4. Where is the supraorbital notch typically located?
   a. At the midpoint of the supraorbital margin
   b. At the junction of the medial one-third with the lateral two-thirds of the supraorbital margin
   c. Immediately above the superciliary arch
   d. At the base of the mandible, near the mental foramen

5. What procedure is shown in the below image?

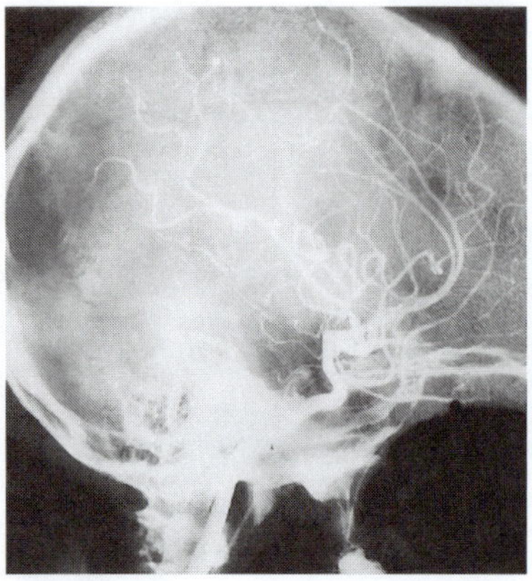

a. X-ray-skull b. CT-brain
c. Carotid angiogram d. MRI-brain

6. What position is typically used to visualise sinuses through X-ray imaging?
   a. Water's position b. Trendelenburg position
   c. Sims' position d. Fowler's position

7. In which condition does cerebral moulding produce a characteristic "silver beaten" or "copper beaten" appearance of the skull?
   a. Hydrocephalus
   b. Raised intracranial tension
   c. Meningitis
   d. Cerebral infarction

8. Identify the X-marked structure.

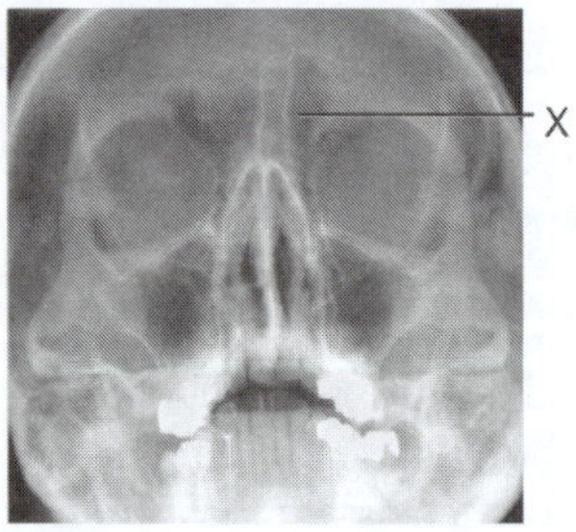


a. Frontal sinus b. Maxillary sinus
c. Nasal septum d. Ethmoidal sinus

9. Identify the X-marked structure.

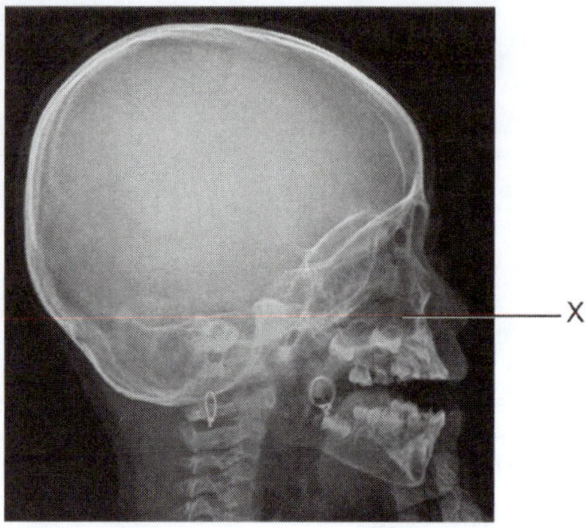


a. Frontal sinus b. Maxillary sinus
c. Nasal septum d. Ethmoidal sinus

10. Identify the surface marking shown in the following figure marked with X.

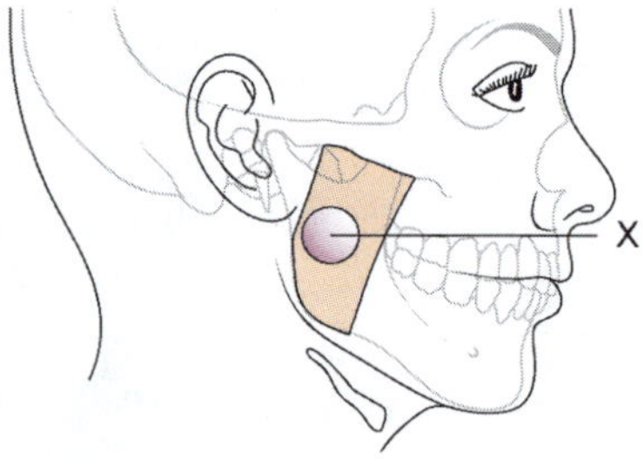


a. Submandibular gland b. Parotid gland
c. Palatine tonsil d. Parotid duct

11. Identify the surface marking shown in the following figure marked with X.

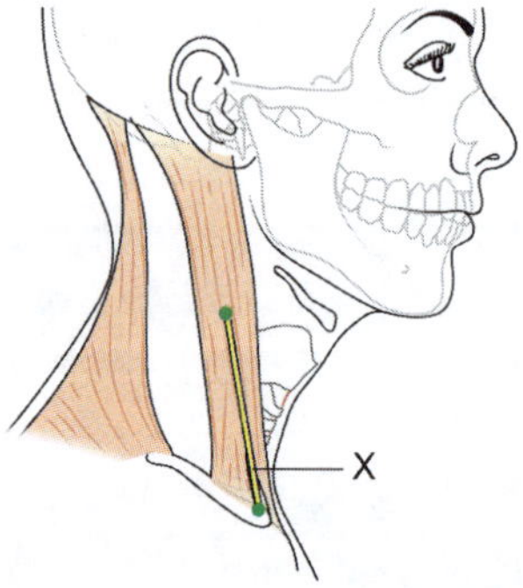


a. Sympathetic chain b. External jugular vein
c. Phrenic nerve d. Vagus nerve

Chapter 1

# Organisation of Nervous System

eSmartQuiz

## CLINICOANATOMICAL PROBLEM

### Clinical Case 1

A 34-year-old man presented with fever, headache, and muscle weakness two months after being bitten by a stray dog. He experienced hydrophobia and confusion. The patient recalled the dog appearing ill and aggressive. Neurological examination revealed signs of encephalitis. Despite supportive care, his condition rapidly deteriorated. **Rabies** was confirmed post-mortem through detection of the virus in brain tissue. The patient's prolonged incubation period was attributed to the bite on his lower leg.

1. How the rabies virus reach the brain in from the lower limb?
2. How the rabies can be prevented?

*Explanation*

1. ______________________________

2. ______________________________

## PRACTICE FIGURE

(Label the practice figure)

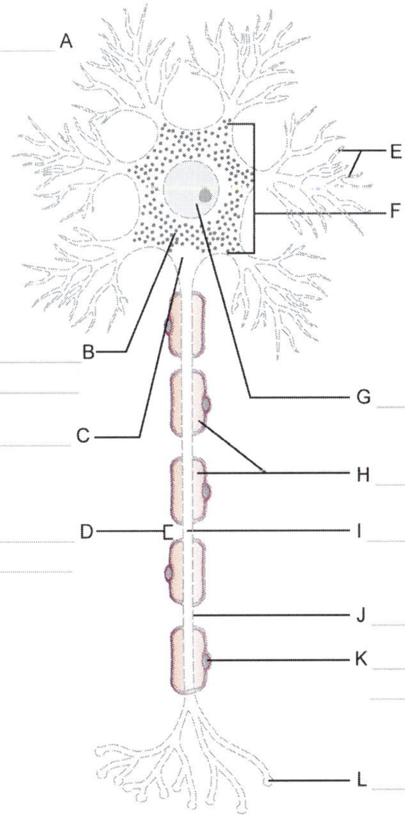


**Practice Fig. 1.1:** Multipolar neuron

## MULTIPLE CHOICE QUESTIONS

(Tick the single best correct option)

1. Pyramidal cells of motor cortex in cerebrum are examples of __________ neurons.
   a. Unipolar b. Pseudounipolar
   c. Bipolar d. Golgi type I
2. Identify the X-marked cell.

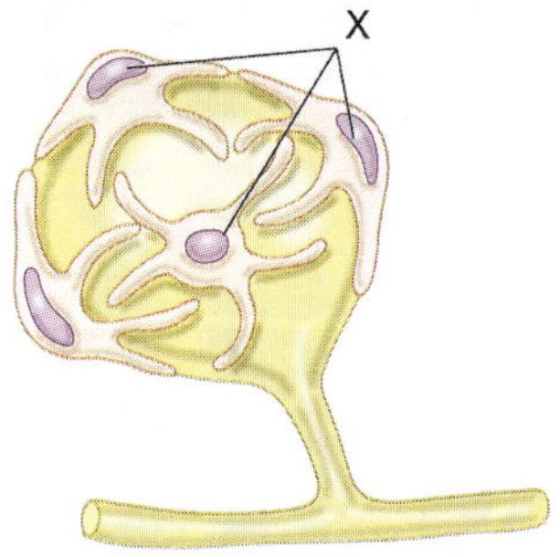


   a. Astrocyte b. Oligodendrocyte
   c. Schwann cell d. Satellite cell
3. How many neurons are present in brain?
   a. 120–140 billion b. 140–160 billion
   c. 160–180 billion d. 180–200 billion
4. Cavity present in mesencephalon is called……
   a. Lateral ventricle b. 3rd ventricle
   c. Cerebral aqueduct d. 4th ventricle
5. All of the following statements is true about axon, EXCEPT:
   a. Axon is a single, long and thin process of neuron
   b. Axons carry information away from the neuron body and have a uniform diameter
   c. Axoplasm is cytoplasm in axon and axolemma is its cell membrane
   d. Axons contain rough endoplasmic reticulum and Nissl granules
6. Which of the following is unipolar neuron?
   a. Dorsal root ganglia
   b. Sensory nerve ganglia
   c. Ganglionic cells of vestibular ganglia
   d. Neurons of mesencephalic nucleus of trigeminal nucleus
7. All of the following are multipolar neurons, EXCEPT:
   a. Stellate cells b. Purkinje cells
   c. Pyramidal cells d. Cells of retina

11. Anterior horn cells of the spinal cord are examples of __________ neurons.
   a. Unipolar
   b. Pseudounipolar
   c. Bipolar
   d. Multipolar

9. All of the following are central neuroglia, EXCEPT:
   a. Astrocytes
   b. Oligodendrocytes
   c. Satellite cells
   d. Ependymal cells
10. Myelination in central nervous system is done by __________.
   a. Astrocytes
   b. Oligodendrocytes
   c. Satellite cells
   d. Schwann cells
11. Cavity present in rhombencephalon is called __________.
   a. Lateral ventricle b. 3rd ventricle
   c. Cerebral aqueduct d. 4th ventricle
12. The spinal segments tested in the knee jerk are:
   a. L1, L2 b. L3, L4
   c. L5, S1 d. S2, S3
13. Blood–brain barrier is absent at:
   a. Area postrema
   b. Basal ganglia
   c. Pineal gland
   d. Intercolumnar tubercle

## QUESTION BANK

(Use separate copy to solve the following question)

Q 1. Write a short notes on:
   a. Structure of neuron
   b. Classification of neurons
   c. Synapse
   d. Classification of neuroglia
   e. Functions of astrocytes

eSmartQuiz

# Peripheral Nerves and Ganglia

## CLINICOANATOMICAL PROBLEMS

### Clinical Case 1

A 27-year-old woman presented with wrist drop and numbness over the back of her hand following a fall on her outstretched arm. She had difficulty extending her fingers and wrist. Examination revealed decreased sensation and weakness consistent with **radial nerve neuropraxia**.

1. What is neurotmesis, axonotmesis and neuropraxia.

#### *Explanation*

1. a. ______________________________

   b. ______________________________

   c. ______________________________

### Clinical Case 2

A 55-year-old man presented with burning pain, tingling, and numbness in his feet, which progressively worsened over six months. He had a history of poorly controlled diabetes. Neurological examination revealed decreased sensation and absent ankle reflexes. Electromyography confirmed **peripheral neuropathy**.

1. What is peripheral neuropathy?
2. Why there is numbness in peripheral neuropathy?

#### *Explanation*

1. ______________________________

2. ______________________________

## PRACTICE FIGURE

(Label the practice figure)

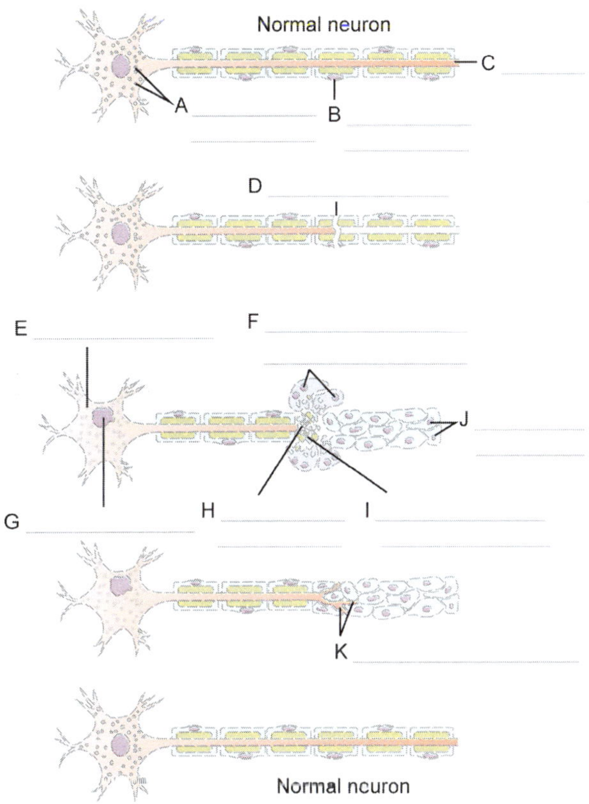


**Practice Figure 2.1:** Degeneration and regeneration of a nerve fibre (Wallerian degeneration)

## MULTIPLE CHOICE QUESTIONS

(Tick the single best correct option)

1. There are __________ pairs of spinal nerve.
   a. 29　　b. 30
   c. 31　　d. 32
2. Which of the following statements about the myelin sheath is NOT true?
   a. Gap between the segments of myelin and between adjacent Schwann cells is called nodes of Ranvier or incisura myelini
   b. Nodes of Ranvier increase the rate of nerve conduction by saltatory conduction
   c. Internode is a segment of myelin sheath between adjacent nodes of Ranvier
   d. Thickness of the myelin sheath depends on the Schwann cell and not on the axon diameter

3. Which of the following statements accurately describes Schmidt-Lanterman clefts?
   a. Schmidt-Lanterman clefts are found in the outermost layer of the myelin sheath
   b. Schmidt-Lanterman clefts contain extracellular fluid between the layers of the myelin sheath
   c. Schmidt-Lanterman clefts are small pockets of cytoplasm in the inner layers of the myelin sheath
   d. Schmidt-Lanterman clefts are gaps formed due to the breakdown of myelin in degenerative diseases
4. In ___________, both axon and myelin sheath damaged.
   a. Neurotmesis b. Axonotmesis
   c. Neuropraxia d. Wallerian degeneration
5. Which of the following statements is true about Wallerian degeneration?
   a. Wallerian degeneration involves the repair of damaged neurons without any degradation
   b. In Wallerian degeneration, only the myelin sheath is damaged while the axon remains intact
   c. Wallerian degeneration occurs in the central nervous system and not in the peripheral nervous system
   d. Wallerian degeneration is the process where the axon distal to the site of injury degenerates along with the myelin sheath
6. Identify the following image.

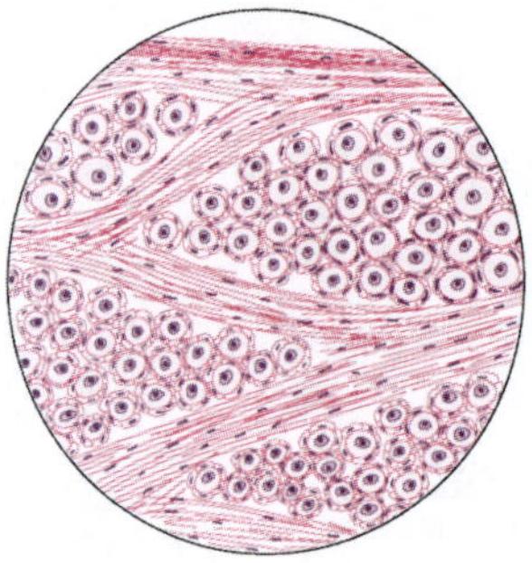

   a. Sensory ganglion b. Optic nerve
   c. Autonomic ganglion d. Spinal cord
7. ___________ involves compression of the nerve root (typical spinal nerve) in case of spondylitis or disc prolapse.
   a. Radiculopathy b. Neuropathy
   c. Myopathy d. Plexopathy
8. ___________ is an autoimmune disease that results in degeneration of the myelin sheath.
   a. Multiple sclerosis
   b. Guillain-Barré syndrome
   c. Chronic inflammatory demyelinating polyneuropathy (CIDP)
   d. Neuromyelitis optica
9. Alpha motor neurons supply:
   a. Extrafusal muscle fibres
   b. Intrafusal muscle fibres
   c. Cutaneous mechanoreceptors
   d. Autonomic ganglia
10. What are vasa nervorum?
   a. Blood vessels that supply nutrients to nerves
   b. Nerve fibres found in blood vessels
   c. Lymphatic vessels in the nervous system
   d. Microscopic nerves within the spinal cord

## QUESTION BANK

(Use separate copy to solve the following question)

Q 1. Write a short notes on:
   a. Structure of the peripheral nerve
   b. Myelin sheath
   c. Action potential
   d. Nerve injuries
   e. Differences between sympathetic and parasympathetic ganglia

# Receptors

eSmartQuiz

## CLINICOANATOMICAL PROBLEM

### Clinical Case 1

A 45-year-old farmer was brought to the emergency room after collapsing in his field. He had been exposed to **organophosphorus pesticides** while spraying crops. Upon arrival, he exhibited pinpoint pupils, excessive salivation, and muscle twitching. Despite immediate administration of atropine and supportive care, his condition deteriorated rapidly. He experienced severe respiratory distress due to paralysis of the respiratory muscles and was unable to be revived. He was pronounced dead shortly after arrival.

Why did the farmer have:

a. Pinpoint pupil
b. Excessive salivation
b. Paralysis of respiratory muscles

### *Explanation*

a. ____________________

b. ____________________

c. ____________________

## PRACTICE FIGURE

(Label the practice figure)

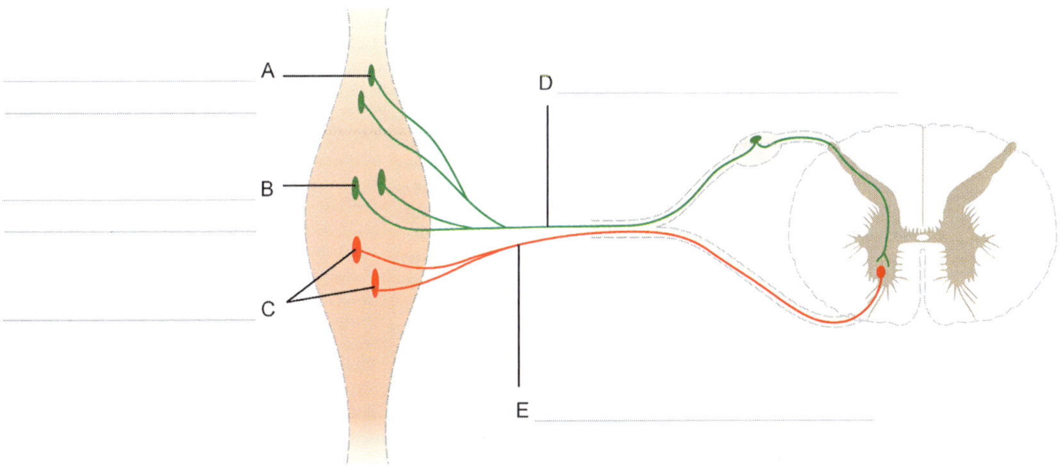


**Practice Figure 3.1:** Stretch reflex

## MULTIPLE CHOICE QUESTIONS

(Tick the single best correct option)

1. All of the following are the type of receptors based on the functional classification, EXCEPT:
   a. Exteroceptors b. Proprioceptors
   c. Chemoreceptors d. Interoceptors
2. All of the following are encapsulated receptors, EXCEPT:
   a. Pacinian corpuscles b. End bulb of Krause
   c. Ruffini's corpuscles d. Merkel disc
3. Which of the following receptor is responsible for torque sensation?
   a. Pacinian corpuscles b. End bulb of Krause
   c. Ruffini's corpuscles d. Merkel disc
4. Identify the following receptor.

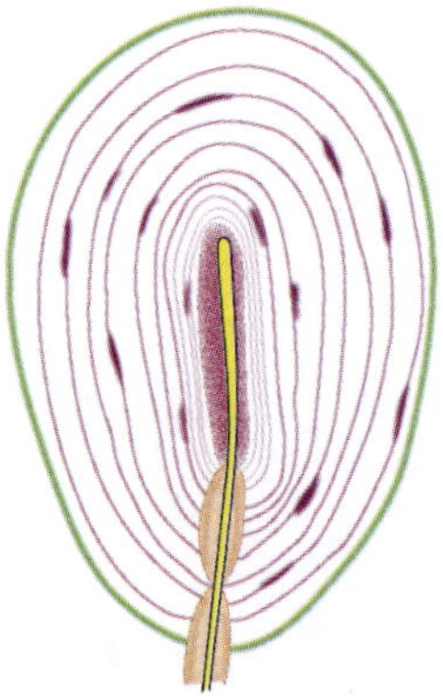

   a. Pacinian corpuscles b. Free nerve endings
   c. Ruffini's corpuscles d. Meissner's corpuscle
5. Which of the following have annulospiral endings?
   a. Type Ia fibres b. Type II fibres
   c. Alpha neurons d. Gamma neurons
6. Which of the following have floral spray endings?
   a. Type Ia fibres b. Type II fibres
   c. Alpha neurons d. Gamma neurons
7. Which of the following is NOT a component of myotatic reflex?
   a. Type I and type II sensory nerve fibres
   b. Muscle spindle
   c. Alpha (α) motor neuron
   d. Dorsal root ganglion
8. In myasthenia gravis, which of the following organ is affected?
   a. Skeletal muscles b. Tendons
   c. Joint capsules d. Bones
9. Identify the structure marked with X.

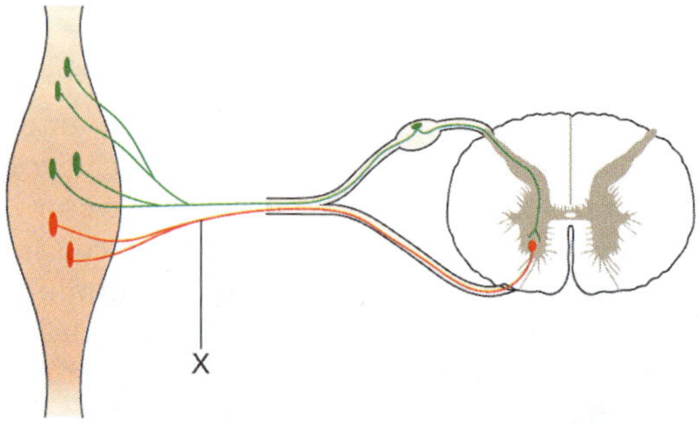


   a. Alpha neuron b. Sensory neuron
   c. Interneuron d. Muscle spindle
10. Identify the mismatched pair.
    a. Meissner's corpuscles – Light touch
    b. Pacinian corpuscles – Deep pressure, vibration
    c. End bulb of Krause – Cold, temperature
    d. Ruffini's corpuscles – Fine touch, heat

## QUESTION BANK

(Use separate copy to solve the following question)

Q 1. Name the various receptors and their functions.

Q 2. Write a short notes on:
   a. Golgi tendon organ
   b. Muscle spindle

Chapter

4

# Meninges of the Brain and Cerebrospinal Fluid

eSmartQuiz

## CLINICOANATOMICAL PROBLEM

### Clinical Case 1

A 6-month-old infant was brought to the clinic with an abnormally large head and bulging fontanelles. The parents reported poor feeding and irritability over the past few weeks. A CT scan revealed significant ventricular enlargement, confirming the diagnosis of **hydrocephalus**. A ventriculoperitoneal shunt was surgically placed to relieve the pressure.

1. What is hydrocephalus?
2. How does the enlargement of ventricles in hydrocephalus lead to an abnormally large head and bulging fontanelles in an infant?
3. What is cisterna magna?

*Explanation*

1. ____________________

2. ____________________

3. ____________________

## PRACTICE FIGURES

(Label the practice figures)

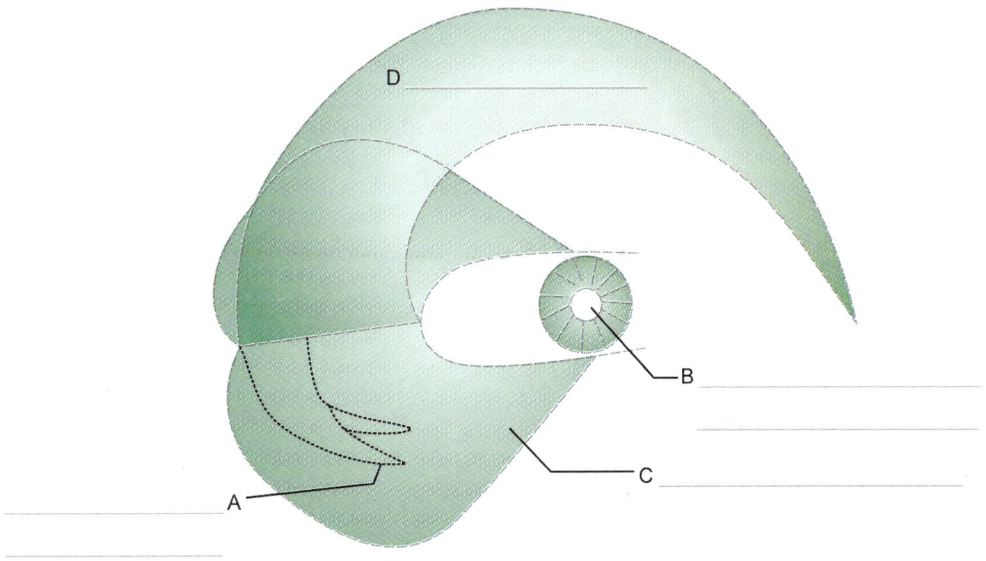


**Practice Figure 4.1:** Various folds of meningeal layer of dura mater

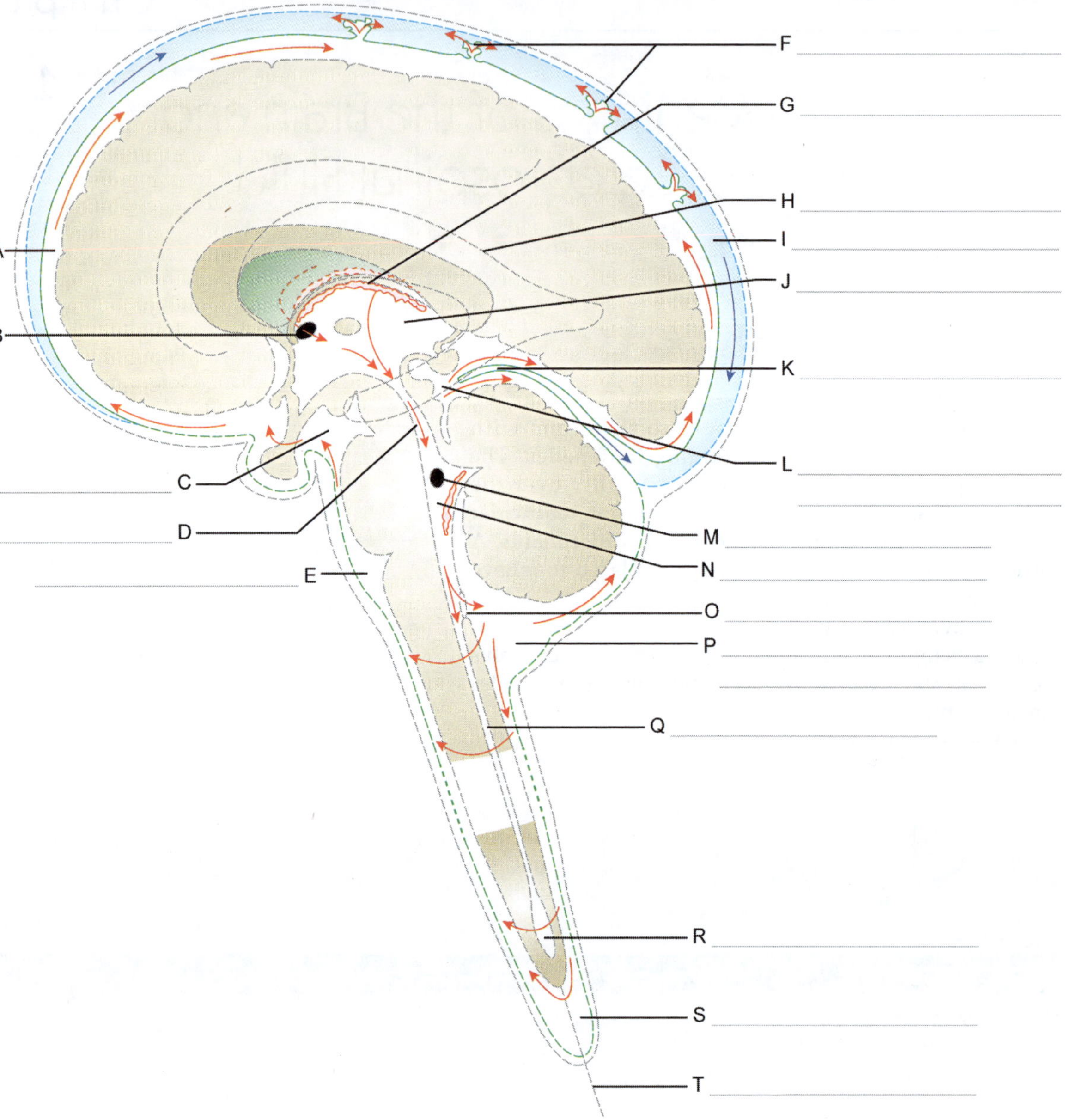


**Practice Figure 4.2:** CSF circulation

## MULTIPLE CHOICE QUESTIONS

(Tick the single best correct option)

1. The space between meningeal layer of dura and arachnoid mater is called:
   a. Epidural space
   b. Subdural space
   c. Subarachnoid space
   d. Perivascular space
2. The space between arachnoid and pia mater is called:
   a. Epidural space
   b. Subdural space
   c. Subarachnoid space
   d. Perivascular space
3. Identify the marked sinus X.

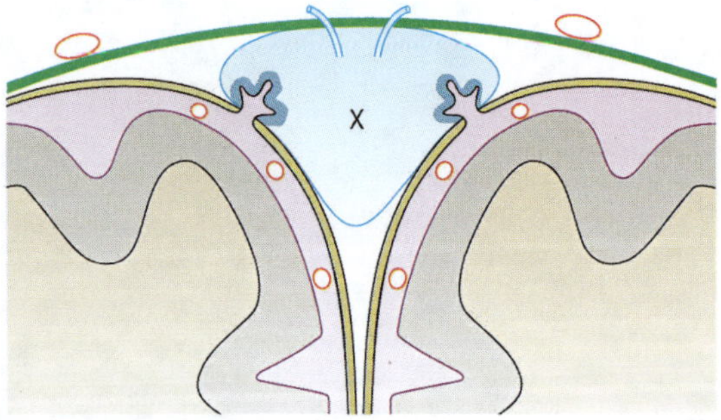


   a. Superior sagittal sinus  b. Inferior sagittal sinus
   c. Straight sinus  d. Transverse sinus

4. Which is the largest CSF cistern?
   a. Cisterna pontis
   b. Interpeduncular cistern
   c. Cerebellomedullary cistern
   d. Cisterna ambiens
5. Which of the following is the anatomical basis of hydrocephalus?
   a. Excessive production of CSF
   b. Obstruction in the circulatory path of CSF
   c. Failure of absorption of the CSF
   d. All of the above
6. Identify the clinical condition shown in the following image.

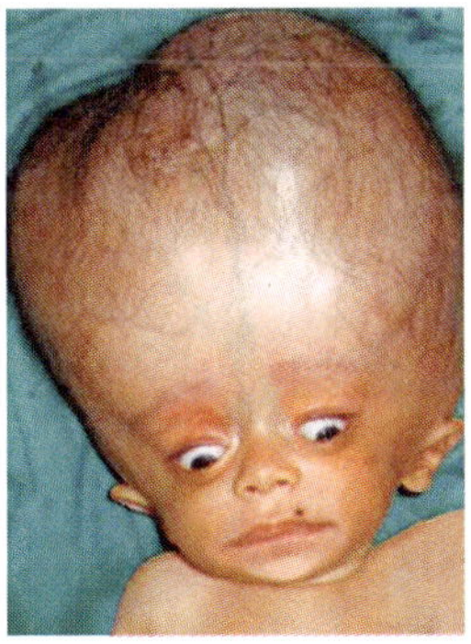

   a. Hydrocephalus b. Capute medusae
   c. Craniopharyngioma d. Encephalocele
7. All of the following are the clinical features of congenital hydrocephalus, EXCEPT.
   a. Disproportionately large size of the head
   b. Enlarged and tense posterior fontanelle
   c. Bossing of the forehead
   d. Setting-sun sign
8. With regards to the arachnoid mater:
   a. It is more collagenous than dura mater
   b. It has two primary parts, the arachnoid barrier layer and the arachnoid trabeculae
   c. The arachnoid trabeculae help suspend the brain in the subarachnoid space
   d. The trabeculae help reduce the weight of the brain by about 97%.
9. The primary enlargement of the subarachnoid space associated with the spinal cord meninges is present in ___________ region.
   a. Cervical b. Thoracic
   c. Lumbar d. Sacral
10. Cerebrospinal fluid circulates around the brain between the:
    a. Skull and dura mater
    b. Dura mater and arachnoid mater
    c. Arachnoid and pia maters
    d. Pia mater and brain surface
11. Which structure connects the third and fourth ventricles?
    a. Cerebral aqueduct b. Interventricular foramina
    c. Foramen of Luschka d. Foramen of Magendie
12. Normally, the total volume of CSF is:
    a. 100 ml b. 150 ml
    c. 200 ml d. 250 ml

## QUESTION BANK

(Use separate copy to solve the following questions)

Q 1. Describe the CSF circulation.

Q 2. Write a short notes on:
   a. CSF
   b. Subarachnoid cisterns
   c. Hydrocephalus

Chapter

# 5

eSmartQuiz

# Spinal Cord

## CLINICOANATOMICAL PROBLEMS

### Clinical Case 1

A 45-year-old male presented to the emergency room following a motor vehicle accident. He exhibited signs of paralysis in lower limbs, with increased muscle tone, hyperreflexia, and weakness predominantly affecting his lower limbs. Neurological examination revealed exaggerated deep tendon reflexes and Babinski sign. MRI confirmed spinal cord injury at the T8 thoracic level.

1. What is the type of paralysis person suffering from?
2. What is Babinski's sign?
3. Why did the patient have increased muscle tone?

#### *Explanation*

1. 
2. 
3. 

### Clinical Case 2

A 55-year-old female presented with sudden-onset severe lower back pain radiating to both legs after lifting a heavy object. She experienced urinary retention and numbness in her perineum and bilateral lower extremities. Neurological examination revealed bilateral lower limb weakness and absent ankle reflexes. MRI showed **compression of the cauda equina** at the L4–L5 level due to a herniated disc. Urgent decompressive surgery was performed to relieve pressure and prevent permanent neurological deficits

1. What is this clinical condition called?
2. Why did the patient have urinary retention?

#### *Explanation*

1. 
2. 

## PRACTICE FIGURES

(Label the practice figures)

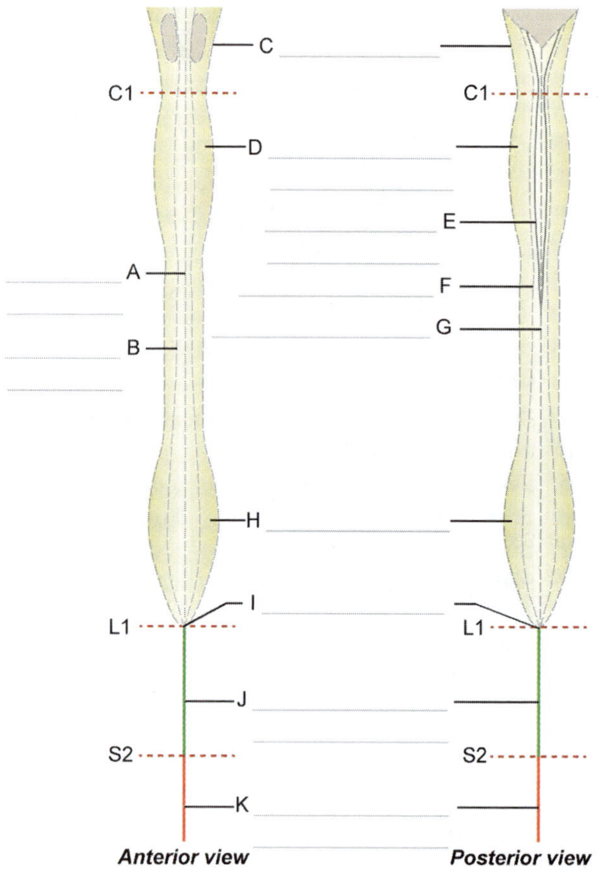


**Practice Figure 5.1:** Extent and external features of the spinal cord

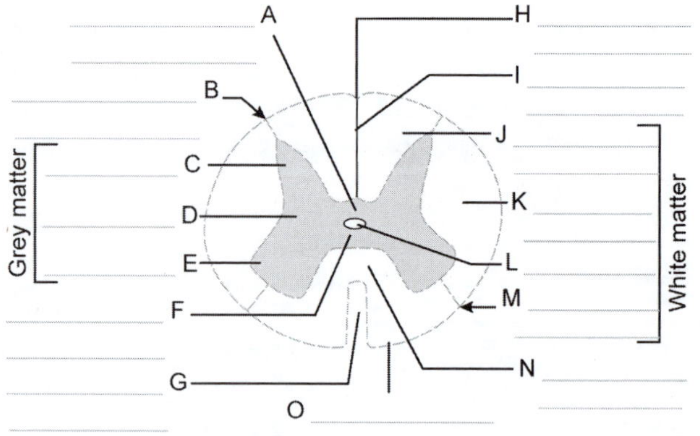


**Practice Figure 5.2:** Transverse section of thoracic segment of spinal cord

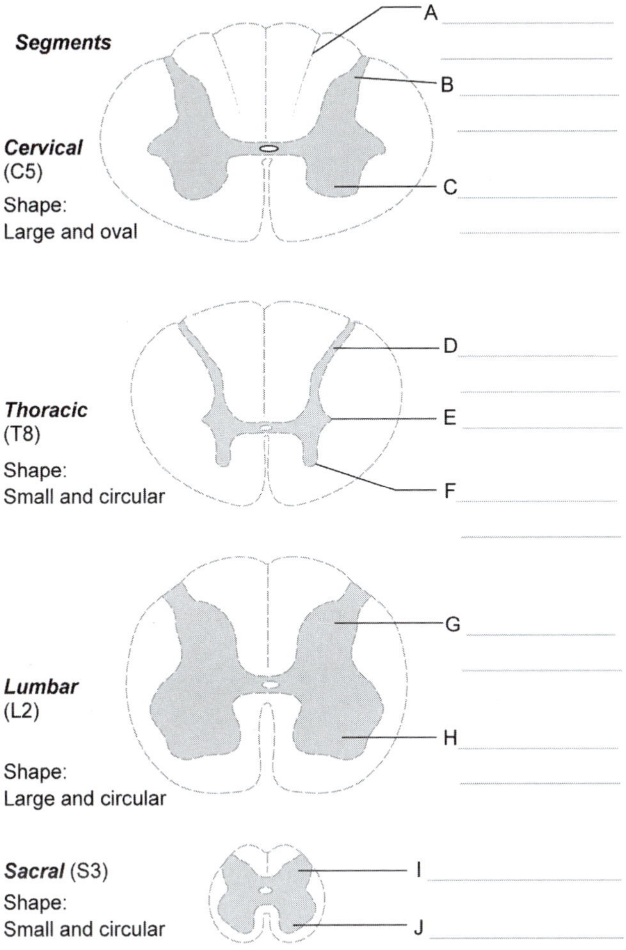


**Practice Figure 5.3:** Features of spinal cord at various levels

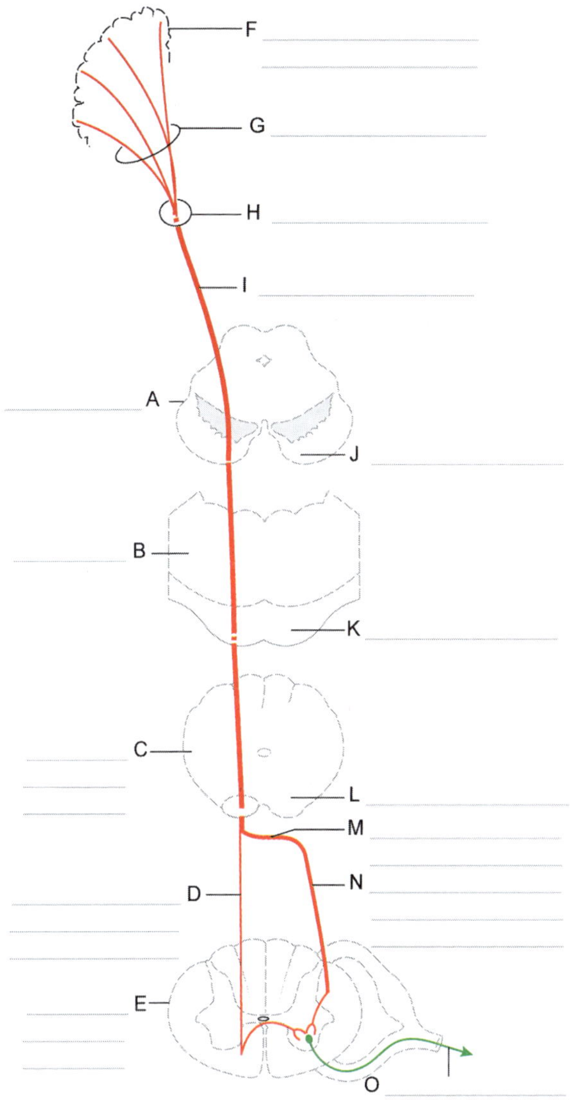


**Practice Figure 5.4:** Pyramidal/corticospinal tracts—course of corticospinal fibres

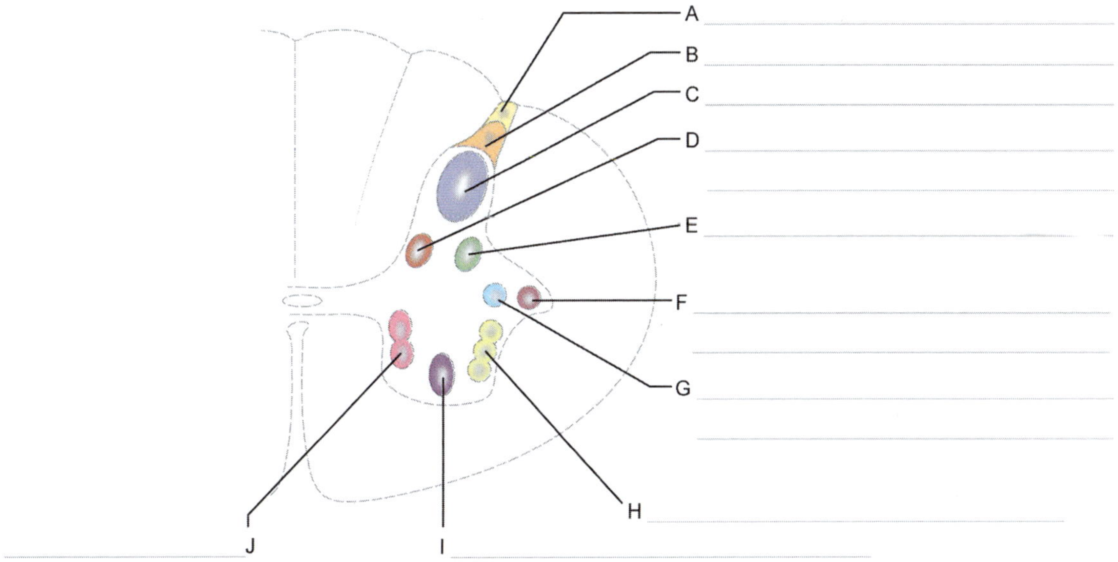


**Practice Figure 5.5:** Cell groups in spinal cord

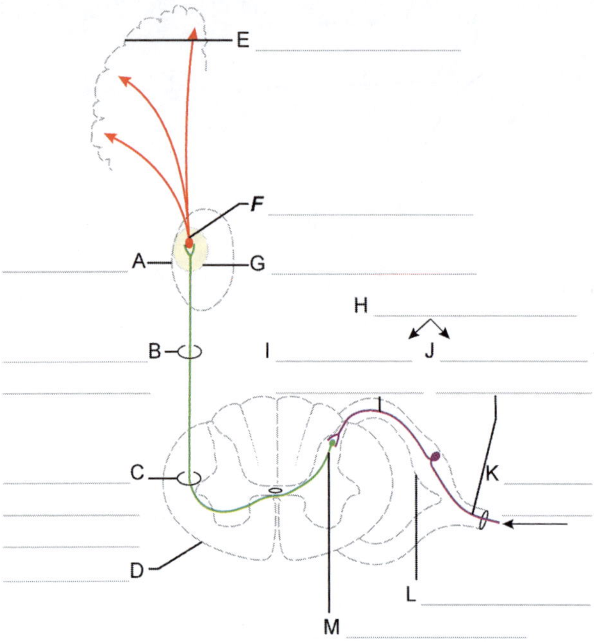


Practice Figure 5.6: Lateral spinothalamic tract

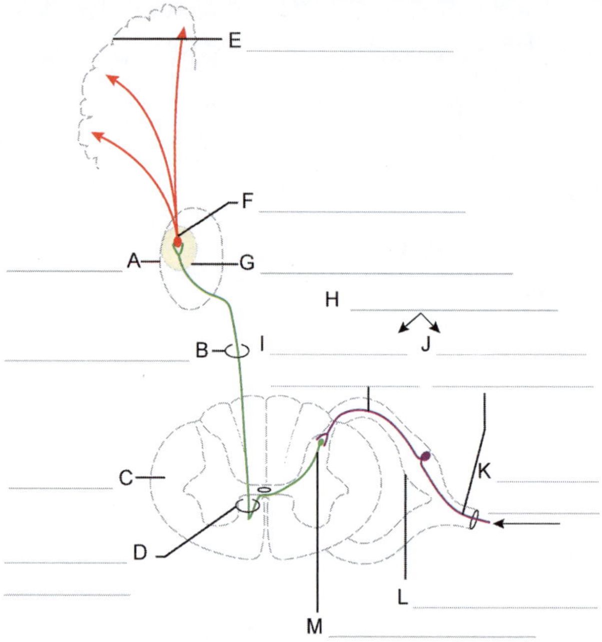


Practice Figure 5.7: Anterior spinothalamic tract

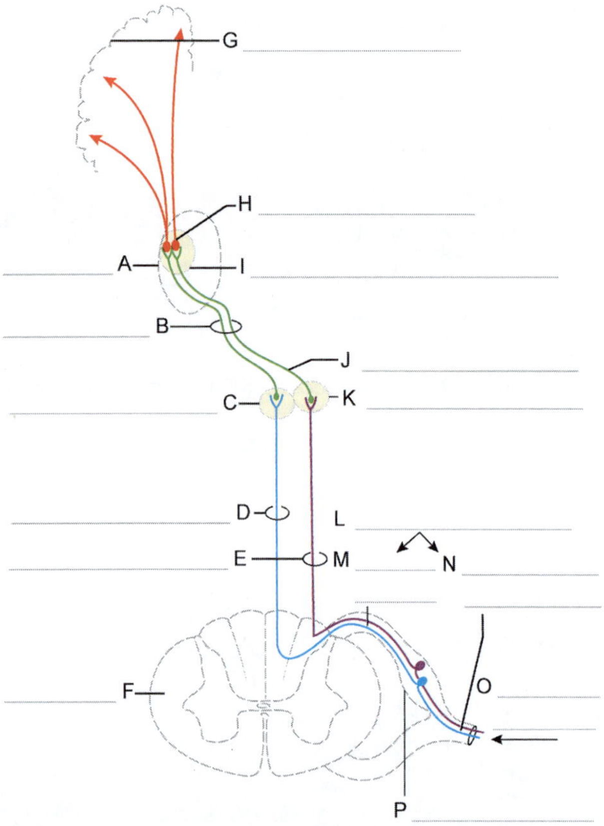


Practice Figure 5.8: Fasciculus gracillis and fasciculus cuneatus

## MULTIPLE CHOICE QUESTIONS

(Tick the single best correct option)

1. What is the lower extent of filum terminalae?
   a. L1 vertebrae
   b. L5 vertebrae
   c. S1 vertebrae
   d. 1st coccygeal vertebrae

2. Identify the following marked tract.

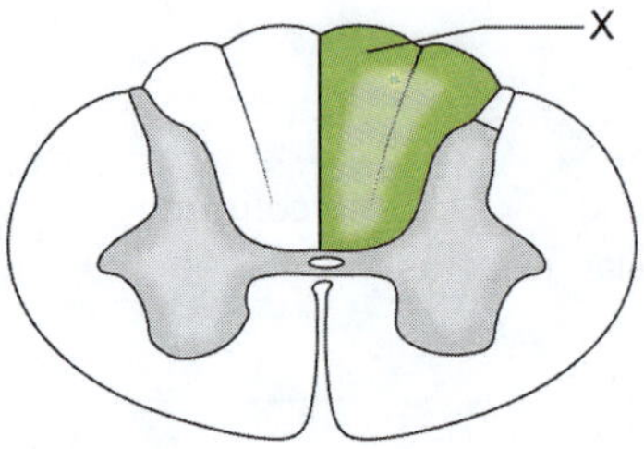


   a. Tract of Lissauer
   b. Fasciculus gracilis
   c. Fasciculus cuneatus
   d. Dorsal spinocerebellar

3. Identify the segment of spinal cord shown below.

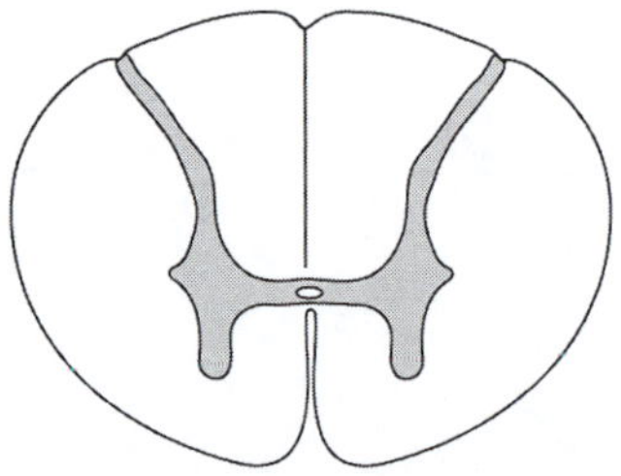

   a. Cervical b. Thoracic
   c. Lumbar d. Sacral

4. All of the following statements are true about cauda equina syndrome, EXCEPT:
   a. Upper motor neuron paralysis of lower limbs
   b. Loss of tendon reflexes of lower limb
   c. Saddle-shaped anaesthesia
   d. Severe root pain

5. Lateral horns of the spinal cord are absent in ____________ spinal segment.
   a. C6 b. T7
   c. L1 d. S3

6. All of the following is true about Renshaw cells, EXCEPT:
   a. These are Golgi type I neurons and located in the posterior horn
   b. They receive collateral from alpha motor neurons
   c. Each Renshaw cell has short axon that terminates on the cell body of same alpha motor neuron
   d. This neuron provides inhibitory feedback to alpha neuron
7. Which neuronal columns of grey matter of spinal cord receive proprioceptive fibres from Golgi tendon organs, and muscle spindle?
   a. Dorsal nucleus of Clarke
   b. Visceral afferent nucleus
   c. Intermediolateral cell column
   d. Nucleus proprius
8. All of the following is true about spinal cord, EXCEPT:
   a. Spinal cord extends through the entire length of vertebral canal up to 3rd month of IUL
   b. Spinal nerves run horizontally and emerge from corresponding intervertebral foramina
   c. At birth, lower end of spinal cord is located at the level of 1st lumbar vertebra
   d. The process of differential growth of spinal cord continues up to the adult life
9. Which neuronal columns of grey matter of spinal cord receive pain, light touch and temperature sensation?
   a. Dorsal nucleus of Clarke
   b. Visceral afferent nucleus
   c. Intermediolateral cell column
   d. Nucleus proprius
10. All of the following are extrapyramidal tracts, EXCEPT:
    a. Rubrospinal
    b. Olivospinal
    c. Lateral vestibulospinal
    d. Lateral spinothalamic
11. Inhibitory cells situated in spinal cord are known as:
    a. Renshaw cells   b. Golgi cells
    c. Purkinje cells   d. Stellate cells
12. Lateral corticospinal tract terminates at:
    a. Clark's column
    b. Substantia gelatinosa
    c. Anterior horn cells of spinal cord
    d. VPM nucleus of thalamus

## QUESTION BANK

(Use separate copy to solve the following questions)

Q 1. Describe the pyramidal tracts.

Q 2. Describe the lateral spinothalamic tract.

Q 3. Describe the tract of Gall and Burdach.

Q 4. Write a short notes on:
   a. Discuss the differences between the UMNL and LMNL
   b. Mention the formation of spinal nerve
   c. Filum terminale
   d. Name the ascending and descending tracts
   e. Tabes dorsalis
   f. Hemisection of spinal cord
   g. Blood supply of the spinal cord.

Chapter

6

# Cranial Nerves

eSmartQuiz

## CLINICOANATOMICAL PROBLEMS

### Clinical Case 1

A 30-year-old male presented with a sudden onset of double vision and a persistent headache. Examination revealed an isolated **paralysis of the right abducens nerve**, causing a medial squint of the right eye. He was unable to abduct the affected eye. Imaging studies indicated increased intracranial pressure due to a mass effect from a large brain tumour.

1. Why did patient have medial squint?
2. Why did the sixth nerve get affected in increased intracranial tension?

### Explanation

1. 

2. 

### Clinical Case 2

A patient with left-sided hemiplegia was unable to move his right eye medially and upwards. There was right eye ptosis and right pupil was dilated and fixed.

1. Which is the cranial nerve involved in this case?
2. What is the site of lesion?
3. Why did patient have dilated and fixed pupil?

### Explanation

1. 
2. 
3. 

### Clinical Case 3

A 60-year-old female presented with sudden onset weakness on the lower right side of her face, difficulty speaking, and mild drooling. Neurological examination revealed right **upper motor neuron paralysis of the facial nerve**, sparing the upper half of her face. She could still raise her eyebrows and close her eyes. MRI confirmed a left cortical stroke affecting the facial nerve's upper motor neurons.

1. Why is the upper half of the face spared in right upper motor neuron paralysis of the facial nerve?
2. How does a left cortical stroke lead to weakness on the lower right side of the face?

### Explanation

1. 

2. 

## PRACTICE FIGURES

(Label the practice figures)

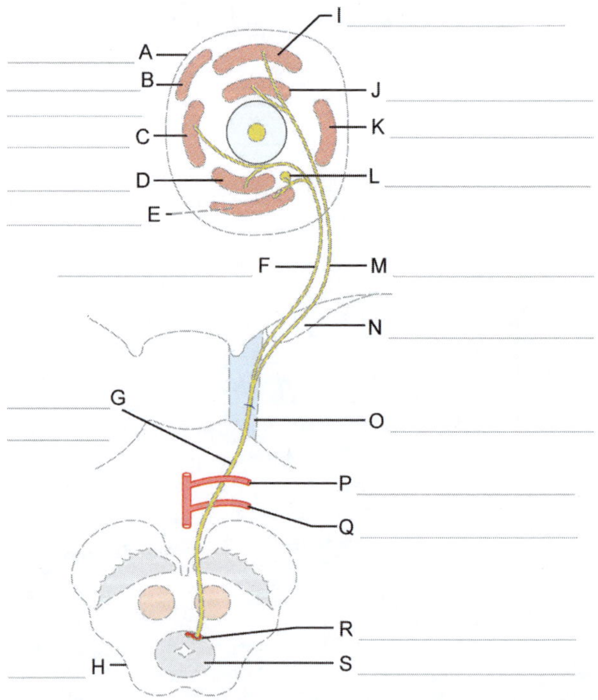


**Practice Figure 6.1:** The origin, course and distribution of oculomotor nerve

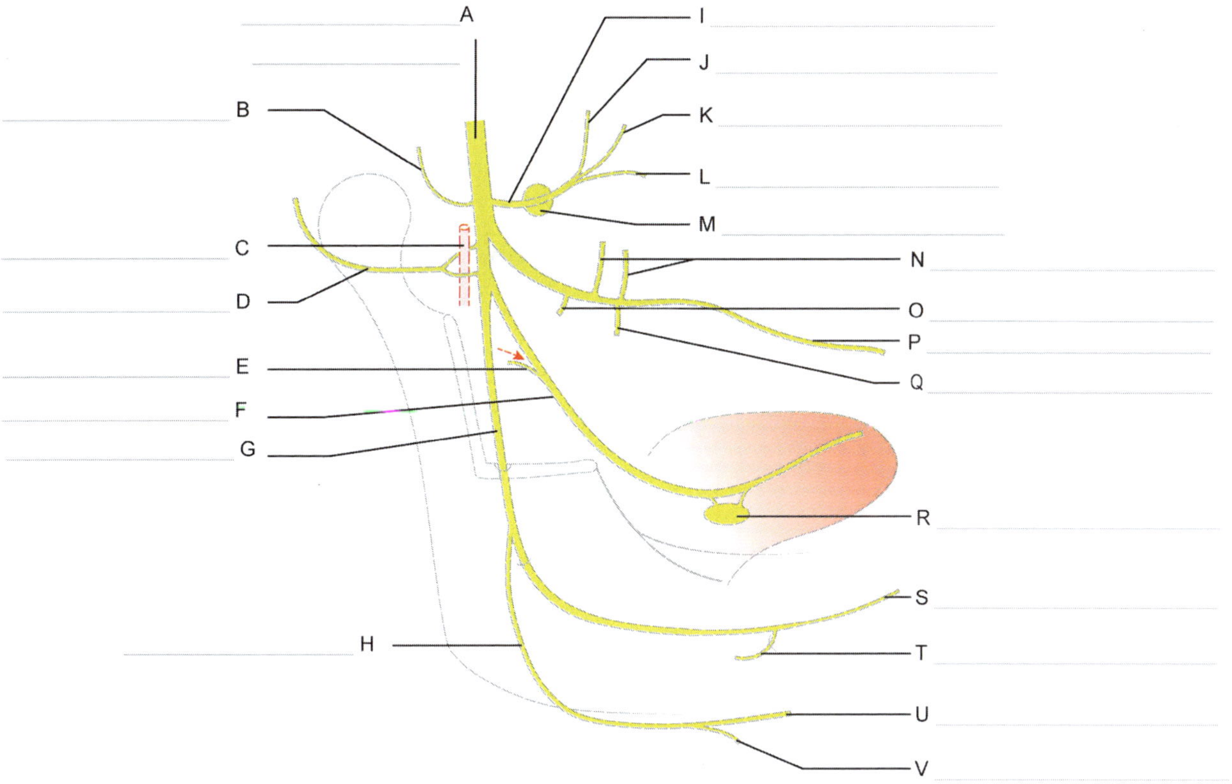


**Practice Figure 6.2:** Course and distribution of the mandibular nerve

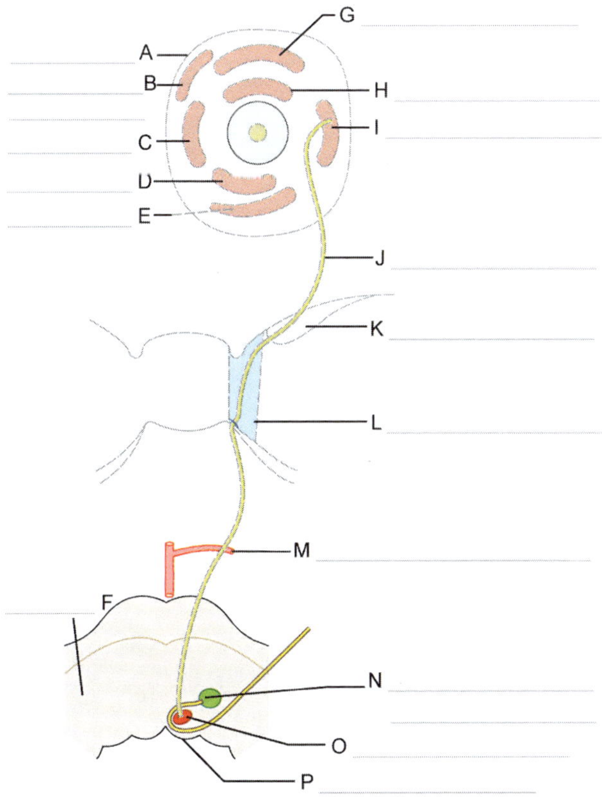


**Practice Figure 6.3:** The origin, course and distribution of the abducent nerve

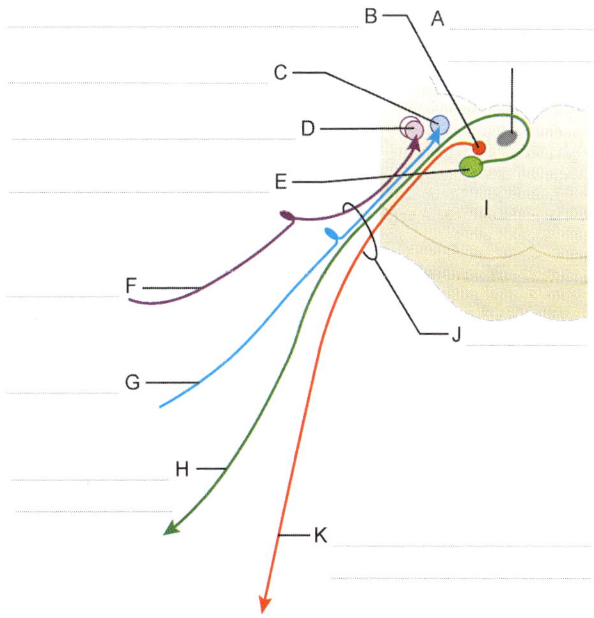


**Practice Figure 6.4:** Facial nerve nuclei

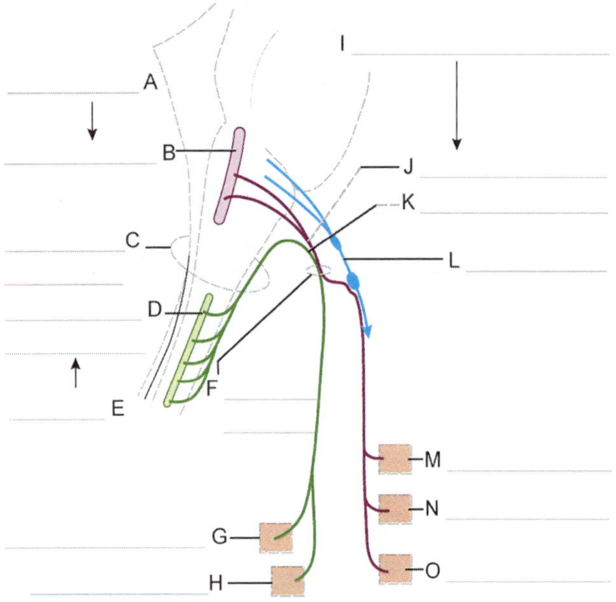


**Practice Figure 6.5:** Course and distribution of the accessory nerve

## MULTIPLE CHOICE QUESTIONS

(Tick the single best correct option)

1. Which of the following is the afferent (sensory) component of cranial nerves that carry taste sensations?
   a. General visceral afferent
   b. Special visceral afferent
   c. General somatic afferent
   d. Special somatic afferent
2. All of the following nuclei of the brainstem carry general somatic efferent sensations, EXCEPT:
   a. Oculomotor nucleus
   b. Abducent nucleus
   c. Vestibular and cochlear nuclei
   d. Hypoglossal nucleus
3. All of the following nuclei of the brainstem carry general visceral efferent sensations, EXCEPT:
   a. Edinger-Westphal nucleus
   b. Nucleus ambiguus
   c. Lacrimatory nucleus
   d. Inferior salivatory nucleus
4. Special visceral efferent fibres from the motor nucleus of trigeminal nerve supply muscles of which pharyngeal arch?
   a. First b. Second
   c. Third d. Sixth
5. Which of the following parasympathetic ganglia are topographically related to the maxillary nerve?
   a. Ciliary ganglion b. Pterygopalatine ganglion
   c. Otic ganglion d. Submandibular ganglion
6. All of the following are branches of the nasociliary nerve, EXCEPT:
   a. Anterior ethmoidal b. Posterior ethmoidal
   c. Supratrochlear d. Infratrochlear
7. Maxillary nerve terminates and continues as which nerve?
   a. Supratrochlear b. Supraorbital
   c. Inferior alveolar nerve d. Posterior ethmoidal
8. All of the following are the functional components of the facial nerve, EXCEPT:
   a. Special visceral efferent b. General visceral efferent
   c. Special visceral afferent d. General visceral afferent
9. All of the following are the branches of the facial nerve, EXCEPT:
   a. Lesser petrosal nerve
   b. Nerve to stapedius
   c. Chorda tympani nerve
   d. Nerve to posterior belly of digastric
10. Which of the following fibres are carried by the chorda tympani nerve?
    a. Special visceral efferent b. General visceral efferent
    c. Special somatic afferent d. General somatic afferent
11. All of the following are the features of Bell's palsy, EXCEPT:
    a. Injury to the facial nerve near or outside the stylomastoid foramen produces Bell's palsy
    b. It is a lower motor neuron type of paralysis of muscles of facial expressions
    c. It may be due to viral infection or unknown cause
    d. It produces paralysis of tongue muscles
12. All of the following features of Patey's faciovenous plane are true, EXCEPT:
    a. It is a plane that divides the parotid glands into large superficial and small deep parts or lobes
    b. Isthmus is a part of glandular tissue that connects superficial and deep parts
    c. This plane is traversed by the trigeminal nerve
    d. In the surgical removal of the parotid gland, care should be taken along this plane
13. Identify the cranial nerve shown in the following figure.

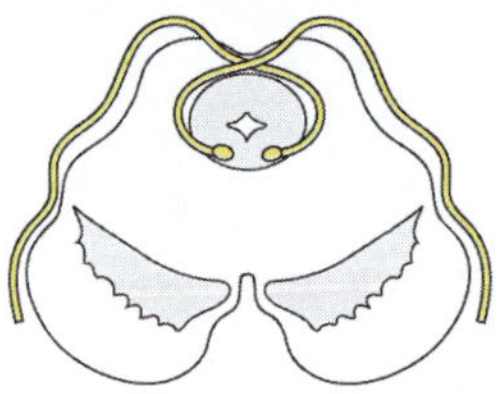

    a. Third b. Fourth
    c. Fifth d. Sixth
14. Ramsay Hunt syndrome is caused by the involvement of the __________ ganglion in the herpes zoster.
    a. Trigeminal b. Geniculate
    c. Submandibular d. Parotid

## QUESTION BANK

(Use separate copy to solve the following questions)

Q 1. Describe the facial nerve and its applied aspects.
Q 2. Describe the hypoglossal nerve.
Q 3. Write a short notes on:
   a. Lesions of visual pathway
   b. Third, fourth and sixth cranial nerves
   c. Mandibular nerve
   d. Glossopharyngeal nerve
   e. Gag reflex
   f. Trigeminal neuralgia
   g. Pterygopalatine ganglion
   h. Otic ganglion
   i. Recurrent laryngeal nerve
Q 4. Describe the following pathways:
   a. Olfactory pathway
   b. Auditory pathway
   c. Visual pathway.

# Brainstem

eSmartQuiz

## CLINICOANATOMICAL PROBLEMS

### Clinical Case 1

62-year-old male presented with sudden-onset right-sided weakness and drooping of the left eyelid. Examination revealed right hemiplegia and left oculomotor nerve palsy. The physician diagnosed it as a case of **Weber's syndrome**.

1. Which part of the midbrain is involved in Weber's syndrome?
2. Which artery is responsible for Weber syndrome?
3. Which structure is responsible for right hemiplegia?

#### *Explanation*

1. ..............................................................
2. ..............................................................
3. ..............................................................

### Clinical Case 2

A 50-year-old female presented with sudden-onset severe headache, followed by rapid deterioration in consciousness. Examination revealed bilateral pinpoint pupils, absent oculocephalic reflex, and hyperpyrexia. Brain imaging confirmed a **pontine haemorrhage**.

Why did patient have: a. hyperpyrexia, b. loss of consciousness, c. pinpoint pupil.

#### *Explanation*

a. ..............................................................

b. ..............................................................

c. ..............................................................

## PRACTICE FIGURES

(Label the practice figures)

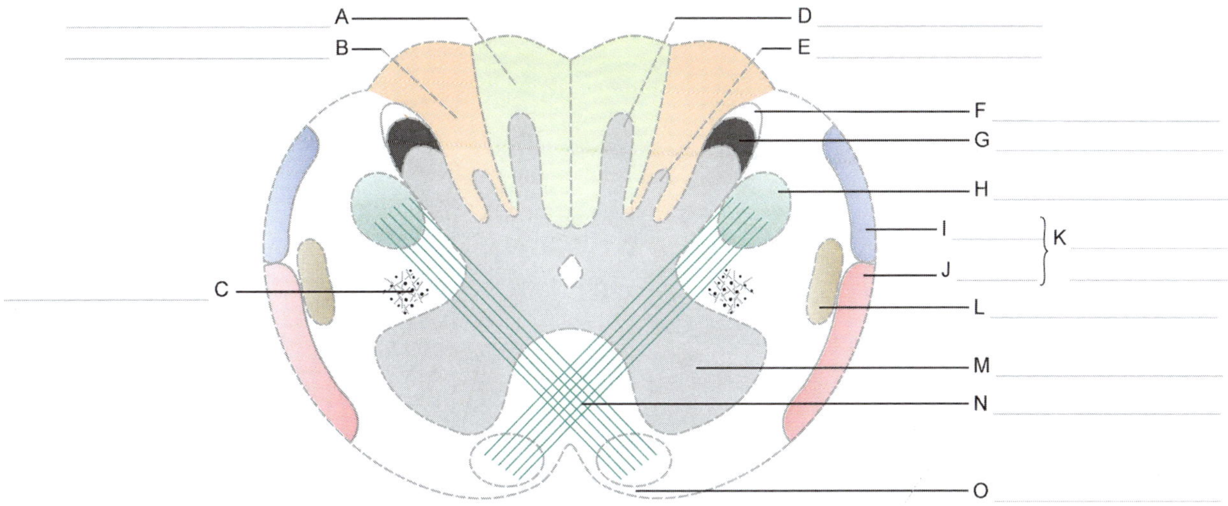


**Practice Figure 7.1:** Transverse section (TS) of medulla oblongata at the level of pyramidal decussation

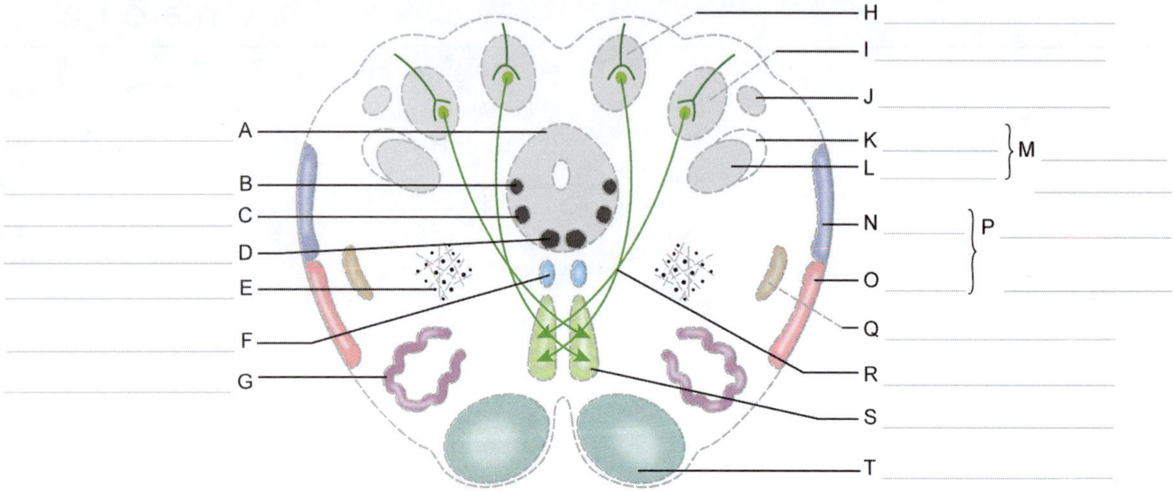


**Practice Figure 7.2:** TS of medulla oblongata at the level of sensory decussation

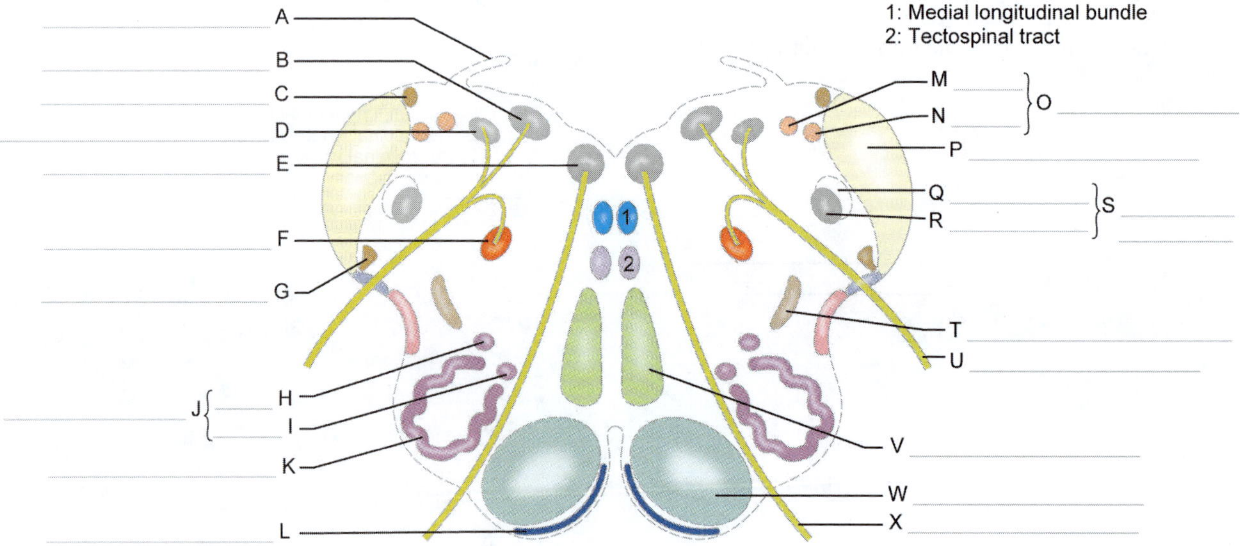


**Practice Figure 7.3:** TS of medulla oblongata at the level of olivary nucleus passing through floor of fourth ventricle

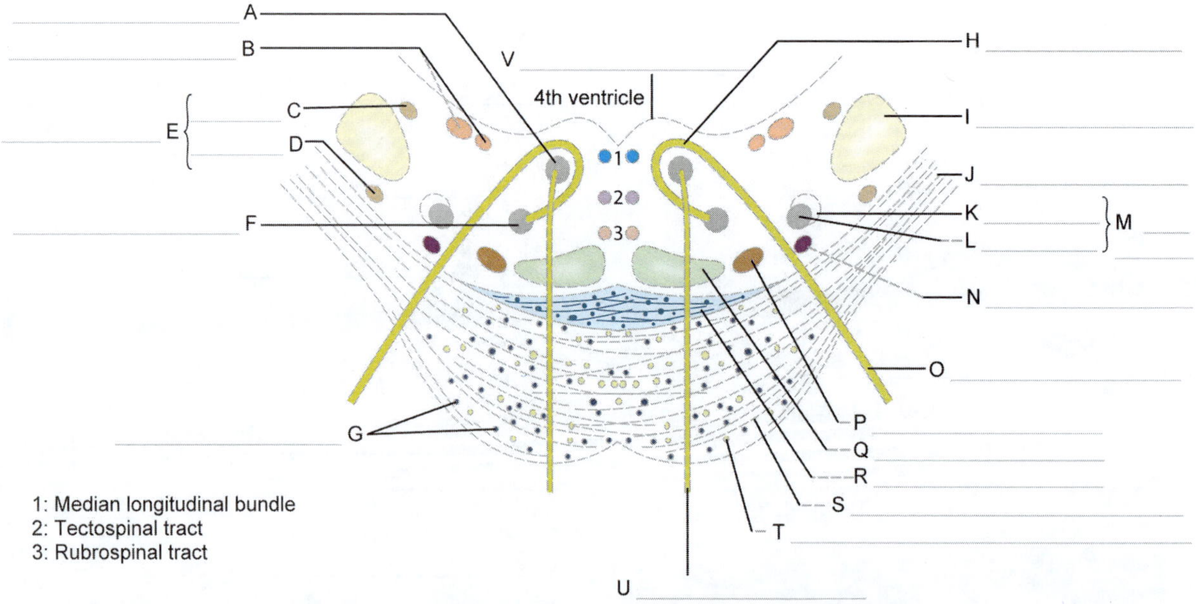


**Practice Figure 7.4:** TS of lower part of pons or TS at the level of facial colliculus

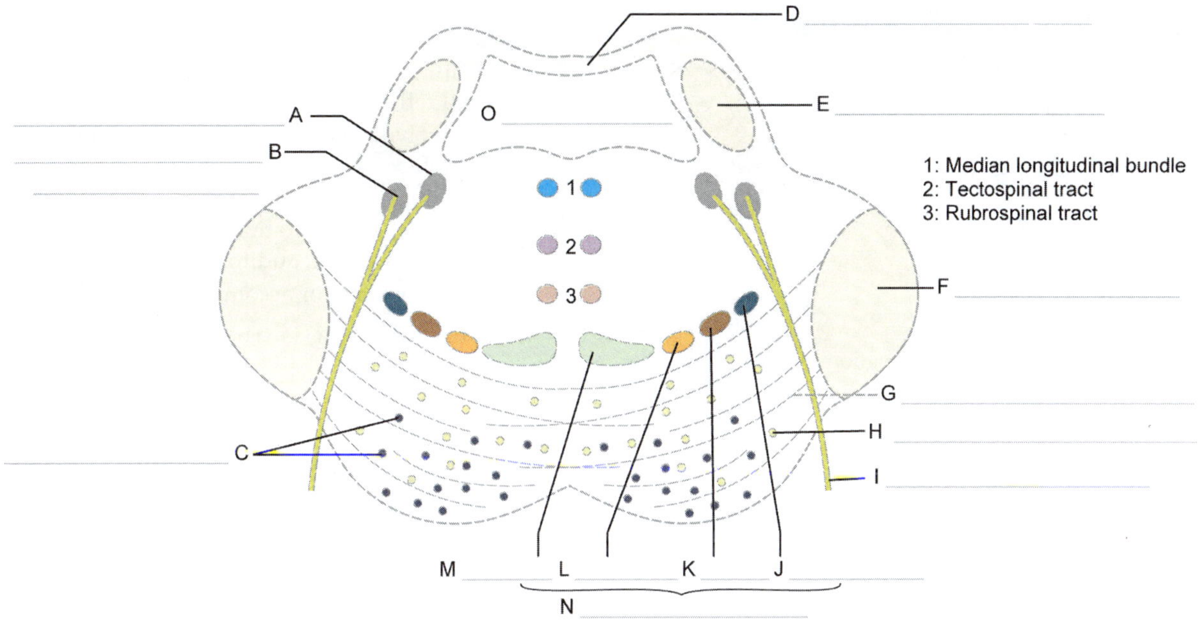


**Practice Figure 7.5:** TS of upper pons

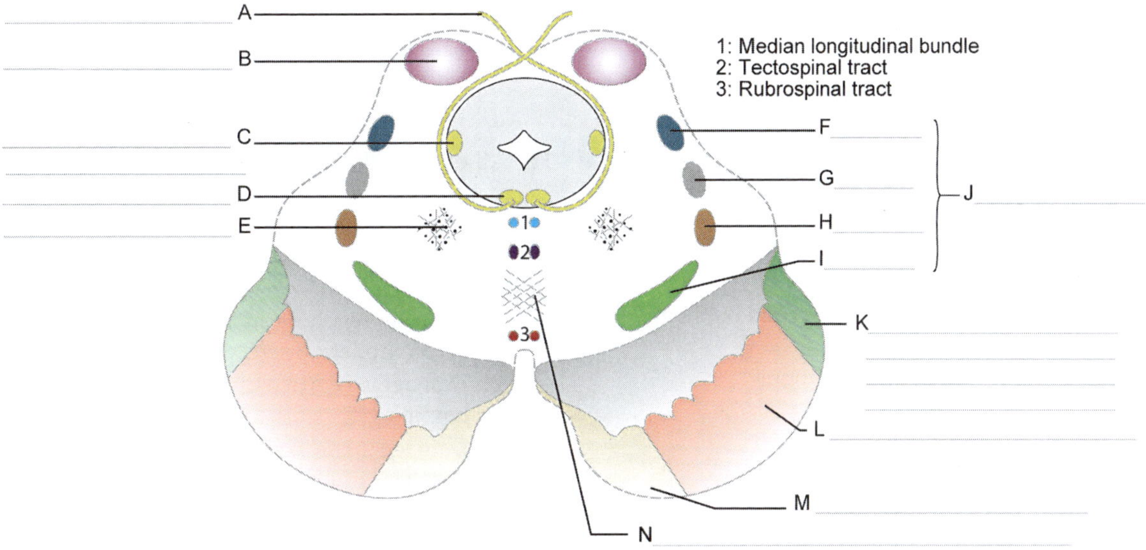


**Practice Figure 7.6:** TS of midbrain at the level of inferior colliculus

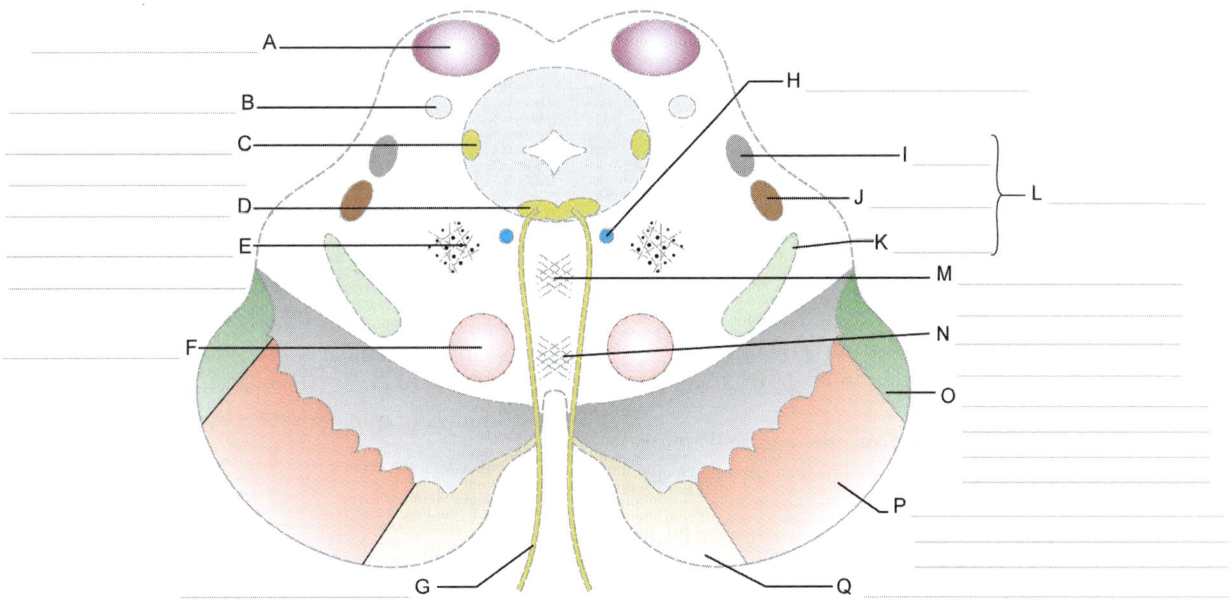


**Practice Figure 7.7:** TS of midbrain at the level of superior colliculus

## MULTIPLE CHOICE QUESTIONS

(Tick the single best correct option)

1. Name the clinical condition resulting from the vascular lesion of the marked red area in following section of the midbrain.

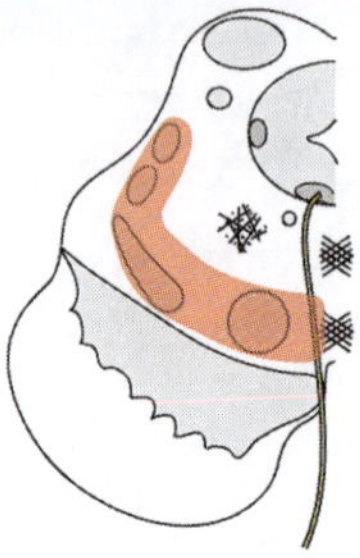

   a. Benedikt's syndrome
   b. Parinaud's syndrome
   c. Argyll Robertson pupil
   d. Weber's syndrome
2. Which nucleus gives rise to preganglionic parasympathetic fibres for parotid glands?
   a. Superior salivatory nucleus
   b. Inferior salivary nucleus
   c. Lacrimatory nucleus
   d. Nucleus tractus solitarius
3. The efferent fibres to the vestibular nuclei comes from all of the following, EXCEPT:
   a. Medial longitudinal bundle
   b. Cerebellum
   c. Spinal cord
   d. Spinal lemniscus
4. All of the following is true about superior olivary nuclei, EXCEPT:
   a. They lie in the anterolateral part of the tegmentum
   b. Most of the fibres of cochlear nuclei relay in the superior olivary nucleus
   c. They form second order neurons of auditory pathway
   d. They primarily process auditory information
5. All of the following sensations are carried by the medial lemniscus, EXCEPT:
   a. Crude touch and pressure sensations
   b. Conscious proprioception
   c. Discriminative touch sensation
   d. Vibration sensation
6. All of the following symptoms are seen in Millard-Gubler syndrome, EXCEPT:
   a. Ipsilateral exotropia
   b. Ipsilateral facial palsy
   c. Contralateral hemiplegia
   d. Ipsilateral loss of proprioception
7. All of the following is true about Foville's syndrome, EXCEPT:
   a. It occurs due to blockage of perforating branch of a basilar artery supplying the dorsal part of pons
   b. Ipsilateral exotropia
   c. Tinnitus, progressive deafness, vertigo
   d. Ipsilateral facial paralysis
8. All of the following is true about crura cerebri, EXCEPT:
   a. The ventral surface of the midbrain shows two crus cerebri
   b. These crus cerebri emerge from the cerebral hemispheres and converge downward at the upper border of pons
   c. They form the posterolateral boundary of the interpeduncular fossa
   d. Trochlear nerve emerges from a groove on the medial side of each crus cerebri
9. Which of the following is the function of pretectal nucleus?
   a. It is associated with auditory pathway and audio–visual reflexes
   b. It is involved in pupillary light reflex and consensual light reflex
   c. It integrates all sensory inputs and generates reflexes such as reflex orientation of eyes, head and neck in response to visual, auditory and somatic stimuli
   d. It is responsible for accommodation reflex
10. All of the following is true about substantia nigra, EXCEPT:
    a. It is a brown-pigmented lamina of grey matter in the pons.
    b. It separates crus cerebri from the tegmentum of midbrain.
    c. It gives rise to dopaminergic nigrostriatal fibres.
    d. All the cells of substantia nigra synthesize dopamine.
11. All of the following nucleus are present in grey matter of transverse section of midbrain at the level of superior colliculus, EXCEPT:
    a. Edinger-Westphal nucleus
    b. Mesencephalic nucleus
    c. Pretectal nucleus
    d. Trochlear nucleus
12. All of the following is true about the features of Weber syndrome, EXCEPT:
    a. Damage to III cranial nerve resulting in ipsilateral lateral squint, drooping of upper eyelid
    b. Damage to III nerve (fibres of Edinger-Westphal nucleus) resulting in dilated pupil, loss of light and accommodation reflex
    c. Damage to corticospinal tract causing contralateral hemiplegia
    d. Damage to corticonuclear fibres resulting in ipsilateral paralysis of lower part of face and tongue.
13. All of the following is true about the features of Benedikt syndrome, EXCEPT:
    a. Damage to oculomotor nerve resulting in contralateral lateral squint
    b. Damage to medial lemniscus resulting in contralateral loss of tactile, muscle, joint and vibration sensations
    c. Damage to trigeminal and spinal lemniscus resulting in contralateral loss of pain and temperature sensation
    d. Damage to red nucleus and superior cerebellar peduncle resulting in contralateral tremors, twitching
14. Which nerve emerge from the anterolateral sulcus, between the pyramid and olive?
    a. Facial
    b. Vestibulocochlear
    c. Rootlets of IXth, Xth, and XIth cranial nerves
    d. Rootlets of hypoglossal nerve
15. Which nerve emerge from the posterolateral sulcus, dorsal to the olive?
    a. Facial
    b. Vestibulocochlear
    c. Rootlets of IXth, Xth, and XIth cranial nerves
    d. Rootlets of hypoglossal nerve

16. Which nerve emerge at pontomedullary junction, above the olive?
    a. 3rd, 4th and 6th cranial nerves
    b. Facial and vestibulocochlear nerves
    c. Rootlets of IXth, Xth, and XIth cranial nerves
    d. Rootlets of hypoglossal nerve
17. The white matter of medulla oblongata shows the following features at the level of sensory decussation, EXCEPT:
    a. Medial longitudinal bundle
    b. Spinal tract of trigeminal nerve
    c. Reticular formation
    d. Spinal lemniscus
18. Nucleus tractus solitarius is a sensory nucleus and receives taste sensation from all of the following nerves, EXCEPT:
    a. Facial
    b. Trigeminal
    c. Glossopharyngeal
    d. Vagus
19. All of the following effects are seen in lateral medullary syndrome, EXCEPT:
    a. Contralateral loss of pain and temperature sensation in trunk and limbs
    b. Ipsilateral loss of pain and temperature sensations over face
    c. Ipsilateral paralysis of muscles of palate, pharynx, and larynx
    d. Contralateral loss of vibration, position sense, discriminatory touch sensation.
20. All of the following effects are seen in medial medullary syndrome, EXCEPT:
    a. Contralateral hemiplegia
    b. Contralateral loss of vibration, position sense, discriminatory touch sensation.
    c. Ipsilateral paralysis of muscles of palate, pharynx, and larynx
    d. Ipsilateral paralysis of muscles of tongue

## QUESTION BANK

(Use separate copy to solve the following questions)

Q 1. Draw a well labelled diagram of the cross-section of:
   a. Medulla at the level of sensory decussation
   b. Medulla at the level of pyramidal decussation
   c. Medulla at the level of inferior olivary nucleus.
   d. Lower part of the pons
   e. Upper part of the pons
   f. Midbrain at the level of the inferior colliculus
   g. Midbrain at the level of superior colliculus

Q 2. Write a short notes on:
   a. Wallenberg syndrome.
   b. Millard-Gubler syndrome.

# Chapter 8

eSmartQuiz

# Cerebellum

## CLINICOANATOMICAL PROBLEMS

### Clinical Case 1

A 6-year-old boy presented with worsening headaches and gait imbalance over 2 months. Neurological examination revealed truncal ataxia and dysmetria. MRI showed a midline posterior fossa mass involving the vermis. Biopsy confirmed **medulloblastoma**.

1. What this syndrome is called?
2. What is truncal ataxia?
3. What is dysmetria?

#### *Explanation*

1. ____________________
2. ____________________
3. ____________________

### Clinical Case 2

A 45-year-old woman presented with difficulty using her right hand and a tendency to sway to the right while walking. Neurological examination revealed impaired rapid pronation and supination of her right forearm, asynergy, intention tremors, and dysarthria. MRI showed a **lesion in the neocerebellum**.

1. What is a. asynergy, b. intention tremors, c. dysarthria.

#### *Explanation*

1. a. ____________________

   b. ____________________

   c. ____________________

## PRACTICE FIGURE

(Label the practice figure)

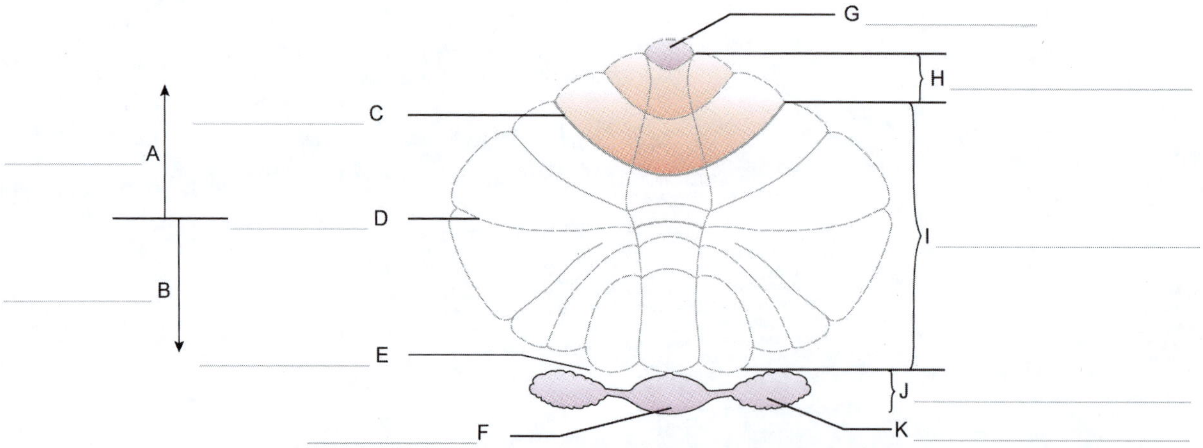


**Practice Figure 8.1:** Lobes, main fissures and surfaces of cerebellum

## MULTIPLE CHOICE QUESTIONS

(Tick the single best correct option)

1. Identify the X-marked nucleus in the cerebellum.

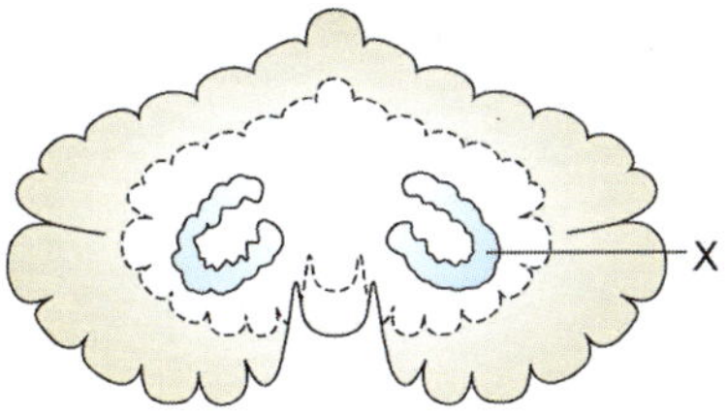


   a. Dentate b. Emboliform
   c. Globose d. Fastigius

2. Which of the following parts of vermis are present in the posterior lobe of cerebellum?
   a. Declive b. Culmen
   c. Folium d. Pyramid

3. All of the following is true about neocerebellum, EXCEPT:
   a. Phylogenetically, it develops last – most recent part
   b. It consists of the posterior lobe expect declive and folium
   c. It coordinates smooth performance of skilled voluntary movements
   d. Neocerebellum is prominent in higher mammals

4. All of the following layers are present in cerebellum, EXCEPT:
   a. Molecular layer b. Purkinje cell layer
   c. Cortical layer d. Granular layer

5. Large flask-shaped cells which arborize in molecular layer of cerebellum is ________
   a. Stellate cells b. Basket cells
   c. Pyramidal cells d. Purkinje cells

6. Climbing fibres of cerebellum are:
   a. Vestibulocerebellar fibres
   b. Olivocerebellar fibres
   c. Pontocerebellar fibres
   d. Spinocerebellar fibres

7. All of the following is true about mossy fibres, EXCEPT:
   a. These are olivocerebellar fibres
   b. They have dilated terminals in granular layer
   c. They synapse with dendrites of granule cells and axons of Golgi cells
   d. This synapse forms light staining cerebellar glomeruli

8. All of the following symptoms are seen in lesion in flocculonodular lobe or archicerebellum, EXCEPT:
   a. Waddling gait b. Disequilibrium
   c. Nystagmus d. Pendular knee jerk

9. All of the following symptoms are seen in lesion of neocerebellum (cerebral cerebellum), EXCEPT:
   a. Dysmetria b. Intention tremors
   c. Nystagmus d. Dysdiadochokinesia

10. Dysdiadochkinesia refers to:
    a. Inability to perform rapid alternating movements with the hands
    b. Inability to stand without swaying with eyes open
    c. Inability to control distance, power or speed of a movement
    d. Inability to perform the tandem-gait test

11. All of the following are functions of cerebellum, EXCEPT:
    a. It initiates the motor activity
    b. Maintenance of posture
    c. Maintenance of muscle tone
    d. Fine coordination of movements

## QUESTION BANK

(Use separate copy to solve the following questions)

Q 1. Describe the cerebellum under the following headings: Gross features, cerebellar nuclei, connections, blood supply and applied aspects.

Q 2. Write a short notes on:
   a. Interior cerebellar peduncle
   b. Nuclei of cerebellum.

Chapter

# 9

eSmartQuiz

# Fourth Ventricle

## CLINICOANATOMICAL PROBLEM

### Clinical Case 1

A 55-year-old man presented with chronic headaches and progressive gait instability. Neurological examination revealed cerebellar signs and **hydrocephalus**. MRI demonstrated an obstructive mass in the fourth ventricle. He underwent surgical resection of the lesion, followed by placement of a ventriculoperitoneal shunt to relieve hydrocephalus.

1. What is hydrocephalus?
2. Why the lesion of the fourth ventricle produces hydrocephalus?

### *Explanation*

1. ______________________________

______________________________

2. ______________________________

______________________________

______________________________

## PRACTICE FIGURE

(Label the practice figure)

## MULTIPLE CHOICE QUESTIONS

(Tick the single best correct option)

1. Inferolateral boundary of 4th ventricle is formed by all of the following, EXCEPT:
   a. Gracile tubercle
   b. Cuneate tubercle
   c. Superior cerebellar peduncles
   d. Inferior cerebellar peduncles

2. Identify the nerve in the given figure of roof of 4th ventricle:

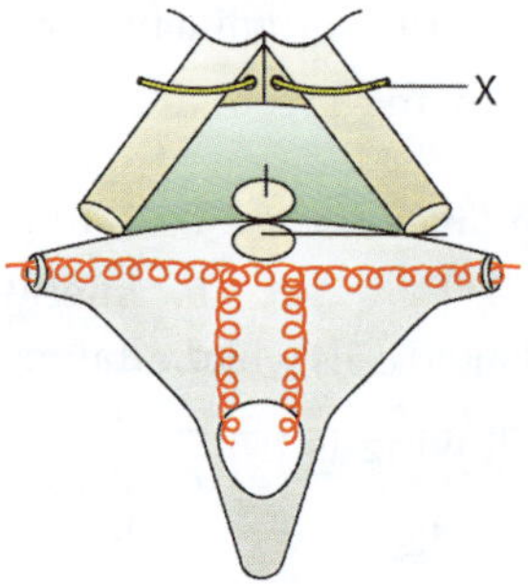


a. Oculomotor b. Trochlear
c. Trigeminal d. Facial

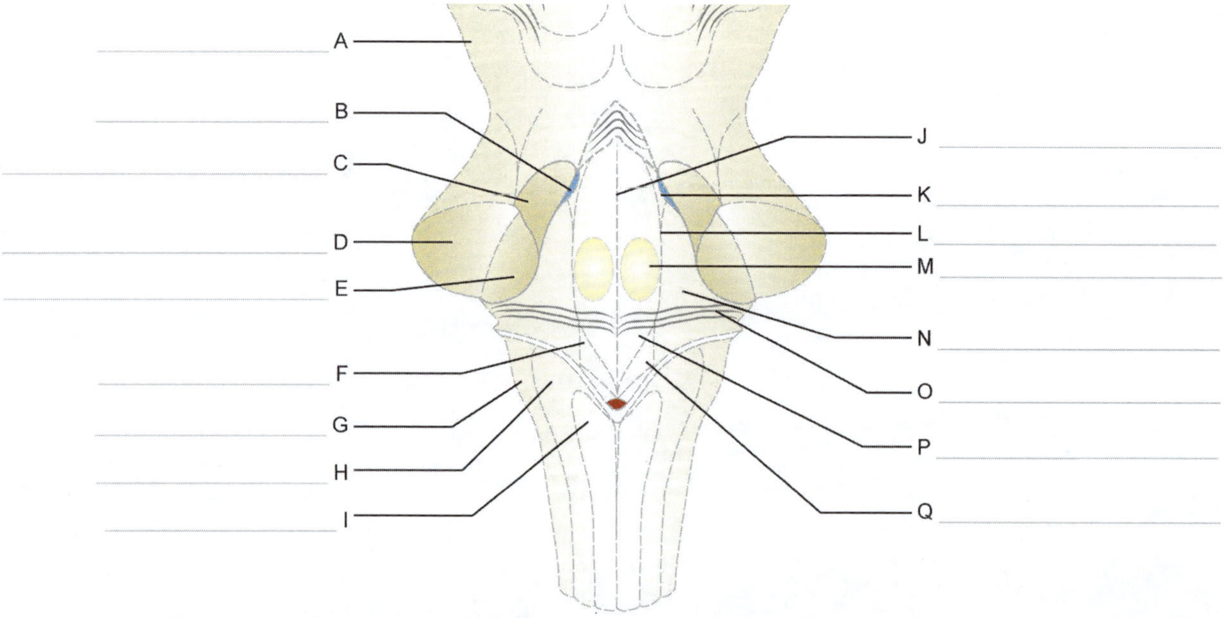


**Practice Figure 9.1:** Floor of fourth ventricle

3. Identify the foramen in the given figure marked with X.

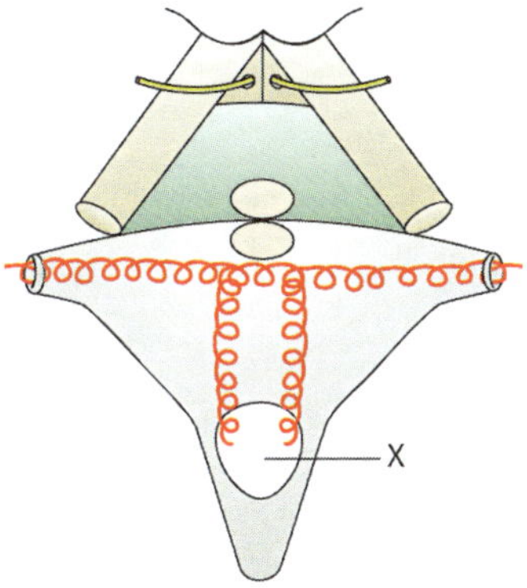


a. Cerebral aqueduct b. Central canal
c. Foramen of Luschka d. Foramen of Magendie

4. All of the following is true about superior medullary velum, EXCEPT:
   a. It is a thin sheet of grey matter
   b. It extends between the two superior cerebellar peduncles
   c. It is triangular, narrow above and wider below
   d. It is continuous with the vermis inferiorly

5. Cavity of 4th ventricle shows all of the following angles, EXCEPT:
   a. Superior angle b. Inferior angle
   c. Medial angle d. Lateral angle

6. All of the following is true about the area postrema, EXCEPT:
   a. It is a small tongue-shaped area
   b. It lies between the funiculus separans above and gracile tubercle below
   c. It contains highly vascular neuroglial cells which act as baroreceptors
   d. It induces vomiting in response to the presence of emetic substances in the blood

7. Identify the marked structure X in the given figure:

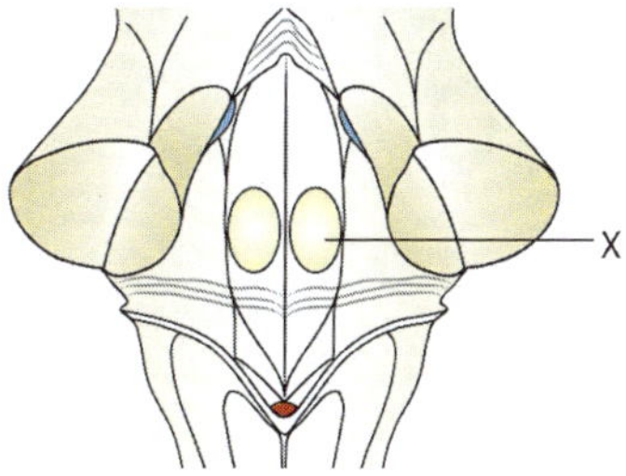


a. Cuneate tubercle b. Inferior colliculus
c. Facial colliculus d. Medial geniculate body

8. The axons of which nucleus are present in the stria medullaris of 4th ventricle?
   a. Gracile nucleus b. Cuneate nucleus
   c. Arcuate nucleus d. Facial nucleus

9. Through which foramen, the 4th ventricle communicates with the subarachnoid space?
   a. Cerebral aqueduct b. Central canal
   c. Foramen of Magendie d. Foramina of Luschka

10. Roof of the fourth ventricle is formed by all of the following, EXCEPT:
    a. Inferior medullary velum
    b. Superior medullary velum
    c. Obex
    d. Median eminence

11. Area postrema functions as:
    a. Chemoreceptor b. Osmoreceptor
    c. Nociceptor d. Exteroceptor

## QUESTION BANK

(Use separate copy to solve the following questions)

Q 1. Describe the fourth ventricle under the following headings: Boundaries, floor, roof, communications, and applied aspects.

Q 2. Draw a well labelled diagram showing the floor of the fourth ventricle.

Chapter

# 10

# Diencephalon and Third Ventricle

eSmartQuiz

## CLINICOANATOMICAL PROBLEM

### Clinical Case 1

A 60-year-old man presented with a sudden onset of severe right-sided burning pain and numbness following a left **thalamic stroke**. Neurological examination revealed sensory loss and hypersensitivity in the right face, arm and leg. MRI confirmed a left thalamic infarct. Despite pain management and rehabilitation, he developed persistent central pain syndrome.

1. Why did patient have: a. sensory loss, b. hypersensitivity.
2. Which is the main artery supplying the thalamus?

### Explanation

1. a. ______

   b. ______

2. ______

## PRACTICE FIGURES

(Label the practice figures)

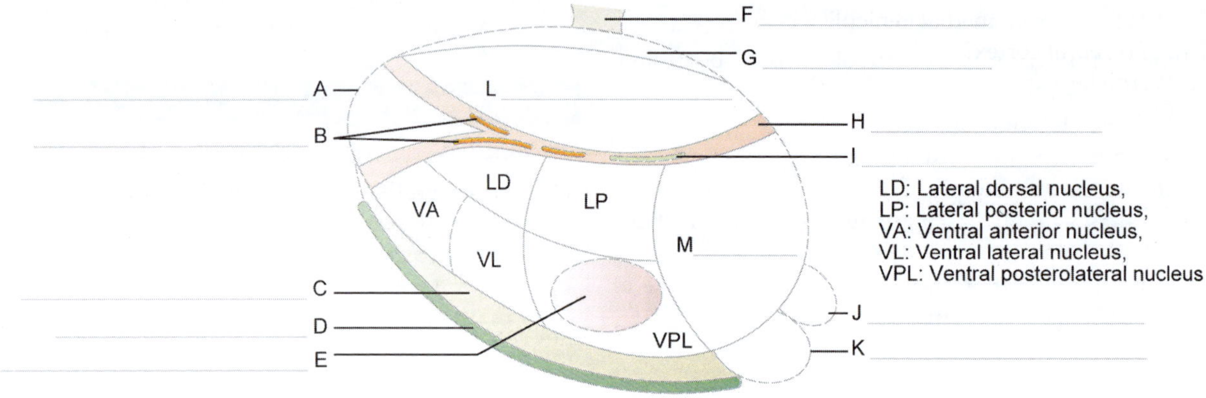


**Practice Figure 10.1:** Thalamic nuclei

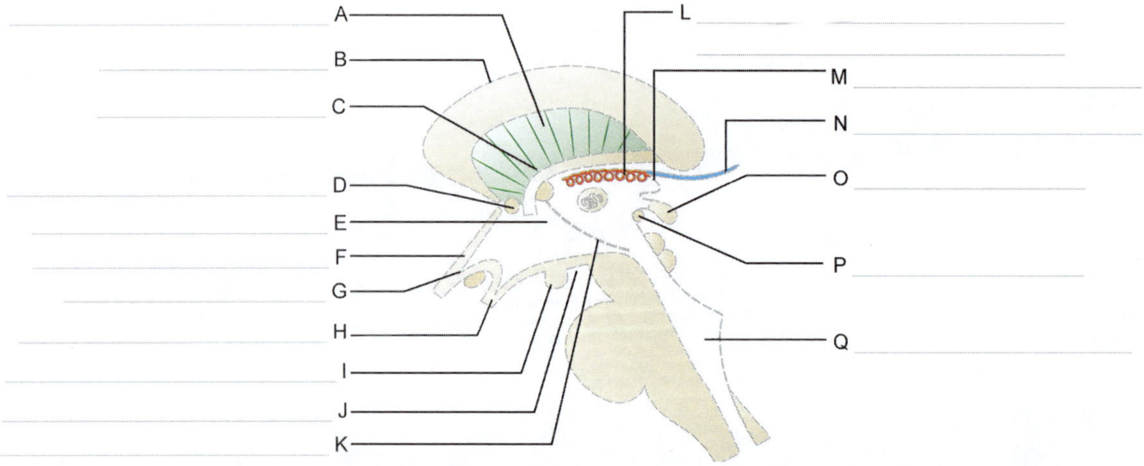


**Practice Figure 10.2:** Boundaries of third ventricle

## MULTIPLE CHOICE QUESTIONS

(Tick the single best correct option)

1. All of the following are parts of epithalamus, EXCEPT:
   a. Pineal body
   b. Habenular nuclei and commissure
   c. Anterior commissure
   d. Stria medullaris thalami
2. Identify the marked structure X.

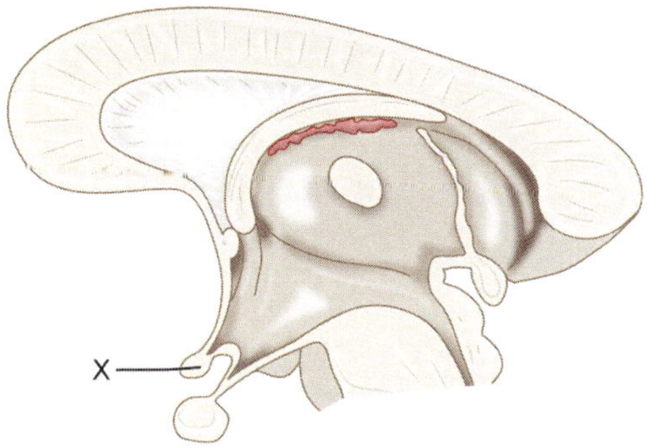


   a. Pineal gland b. Pituitary gland
   c. Optic chiasma d. Anterior commissure
3. Anterior nucleus of thalamus receives afferent fibres from:
   a. Hypothalamus b. Superior colliculus
   c. Cerebellum d. Mammillary body
4. Afferent fibres to medial geniculate body come from:
   a. Substantia nigra b. Inferior colliculus
   c. Pretectal nucleus d. Red nucleus
5. Efferent fibres from medial geniculate body go to which area of cerebral cortex?
   a. Wernicke's area b. Visual area
   c. Broca's area d. Auditory area
6. All of the following is true about lateral geniculate body, EXCEPT:
   a. It is an oval prominence at the posterior end of optic tract
   b. It lies on the inferolateral aspect of pulvinar
   c. It receives afferent fibres from inferior colliculus through inferior branchium
   d. Its neurons are arranged in 6 layers separated by nerve fibres
7. Corpora arenacea is a characteristic feature of:
   a. Pituitary gland b. Pineal gland
   c. Suprarenal gland d. Parathyroid gland
8. Stria medullaris thalami connects habenular nuclei with all of the following structures, EXCEPT:
   a. Septal nucleus b. Basal nuclei of Meynert
   c. Thalamus d. Hypothalamus
9. __________ is a thin layer of grey matter between the subthalamic nucleus and thalamus.
   a. Fasciculus retroflexes b. Fasciculus lenticularis
   c. Zona incerta d. Thalamic fasciculus
10. Which of the following fibres connects medial olfactory area to the preoptic and lateral nuclei of hypothalamus?
    a. Fornix
    b. Stria terminalis
    c. Mammillary peduncle
    d. Medial forebrain bundle
11. Which of the following fibres connects hippocampus to mammillary body?
    a. Fornix b. Stria terminalis
    c. Mammillary peduncle d. Medial forebrain bundle
12. Which of the following nuclei of hypothalamus produces ADH and oxytocin?
    a. Preoptic b. Supraoptic
    c. Paraventricular d. Anterior
13. Which of the following nuclei of hypothalamus is a satiety and hunger centre?
    a. Preoptic b. Supraoptic
    c. Paraventricular d. Ventromedial
14. Which of the following nuclei of hypothalamus is a feeding centre?
    a. Preoptic b. Lateral
    c. Paraventricular d. Ventromedial
15. All of the following are symptoms of hypothalamic disorders, EXCEPT:
    a. Diabetes mellitus
    b. Loss of sexual desires
    c. Polydipsia and polyuria
    d. Aggressive behaviour, rage, or extreme passivity
16. Which of the following do not form the anterior wall of third ventricle?
    a. Anterior column of fornix
    b. Anterior commissure
    c. Habenular commissure
    d. Lamina terminalis

## QUESTION BANK

(Use separate copy to solve the following question)

Q 1. Write a short notes on:
   a. Nuclei of thalamus
   b. Anterior nucleus of thalamus
   c. Hypothalamus
   d. Mamillary body
   e. Nuclei of hypothalamus
   f. Lateral geniculate body.

Chapter

# 11

# Cerebrum, Basal Nuclei and White Matter

eSmartQuiz

## CLINICOANATOMICAL PROBLEM

### Clinical Case 1

A 65-year-old man presented with a six-month history of progressive resting tremor, bradykinesia, and rigidity. Neurological examination revealed a stooped posture and shuffling gait. MRI showed a lesion in the basal ganglia. The patient was diagnosed with **Parkinson's disease.**

1. What is bradykinesia?
2. What is rigidity?
3. Which neurotransmitter is depleted in Parkinson's disease?

***Explanation***

1. ______________________________
2. ______________________________
3. ______________________________

## PRACTICE FIGURES

(Label the practice figures)

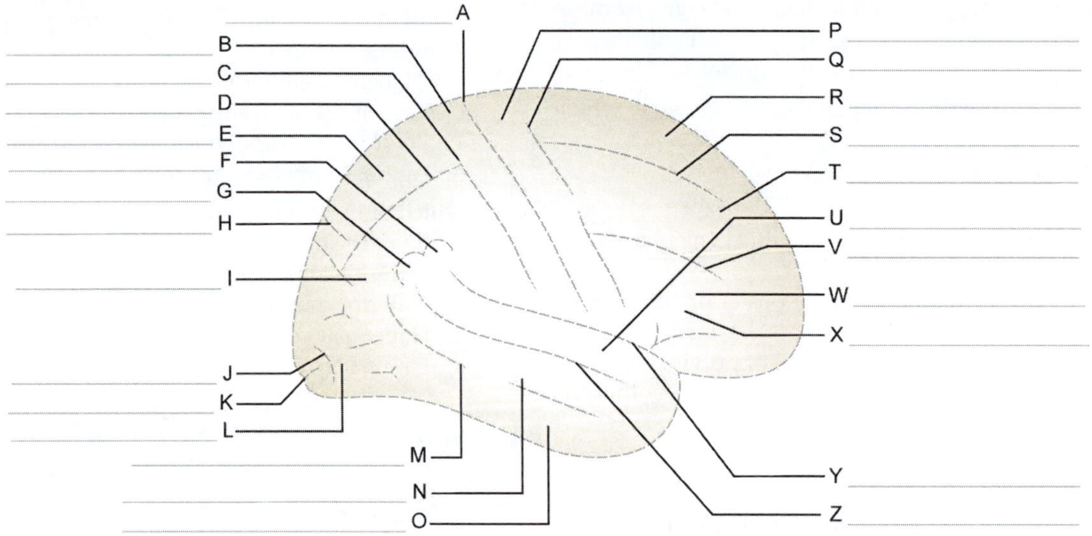


**Practice Figure 11.1:** Sulci and gyri on superolateral surface of cerebral hemisphere

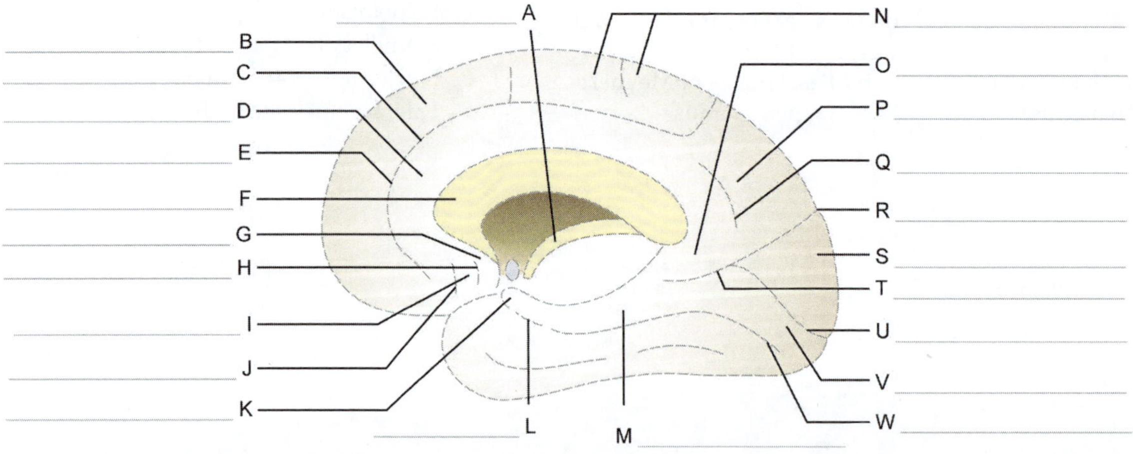


**Practice Figure 11.2:** Sulci and gyri on the medial surface of cerebral hemisphere

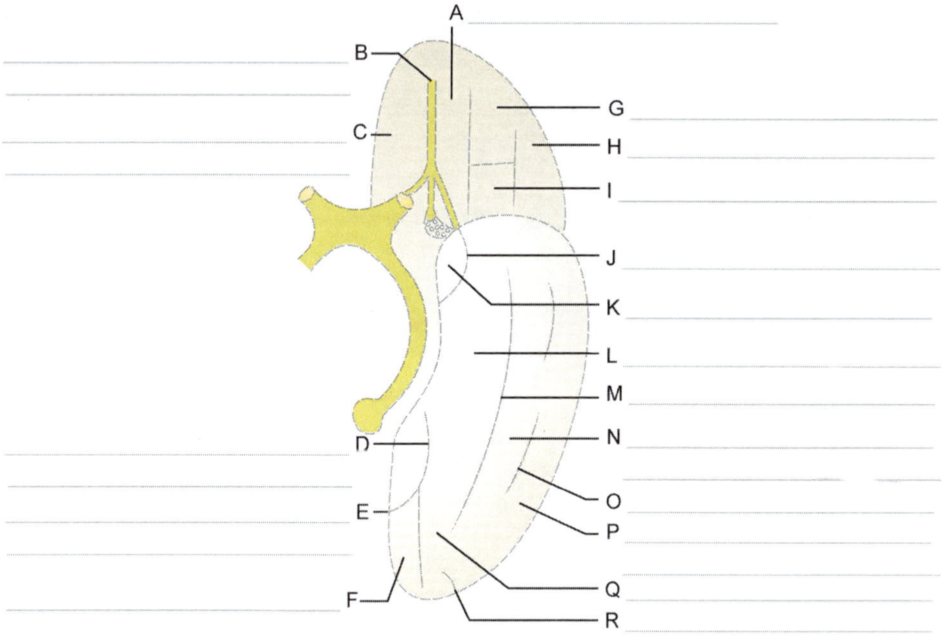


**Practice Figure 11.3:** Gyri and sulci on the inferior aspect of cerebral hemisphere

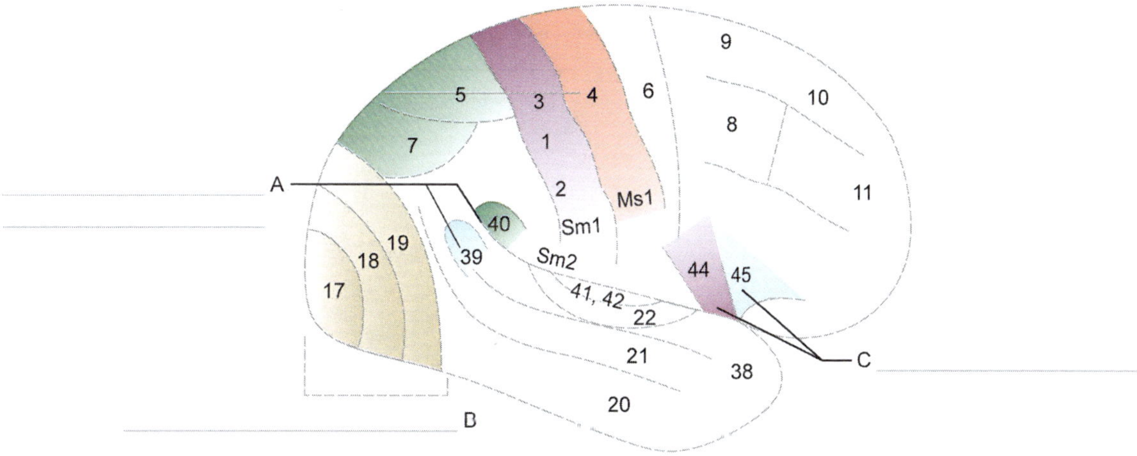


**Practice Figure 11.4:** Functional areas of the superolateral surface of cerebral hemisphere

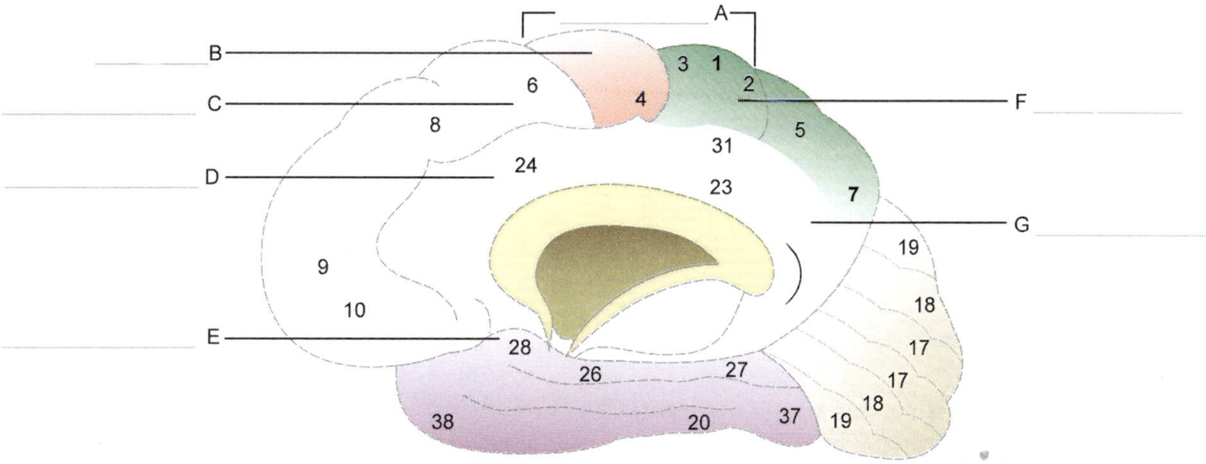


**Practice Figure 11.5:** Functional areas of the medial surface of cerebral hemisphere

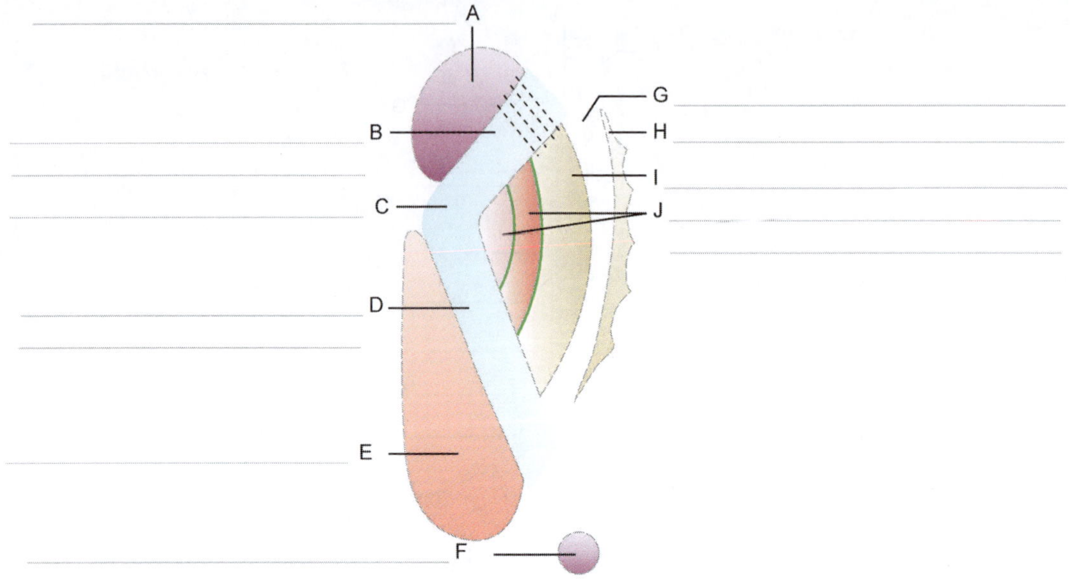


**Practice Figure 11.6:** Horizontal section through corpus striatum, thalamus and internal capsule

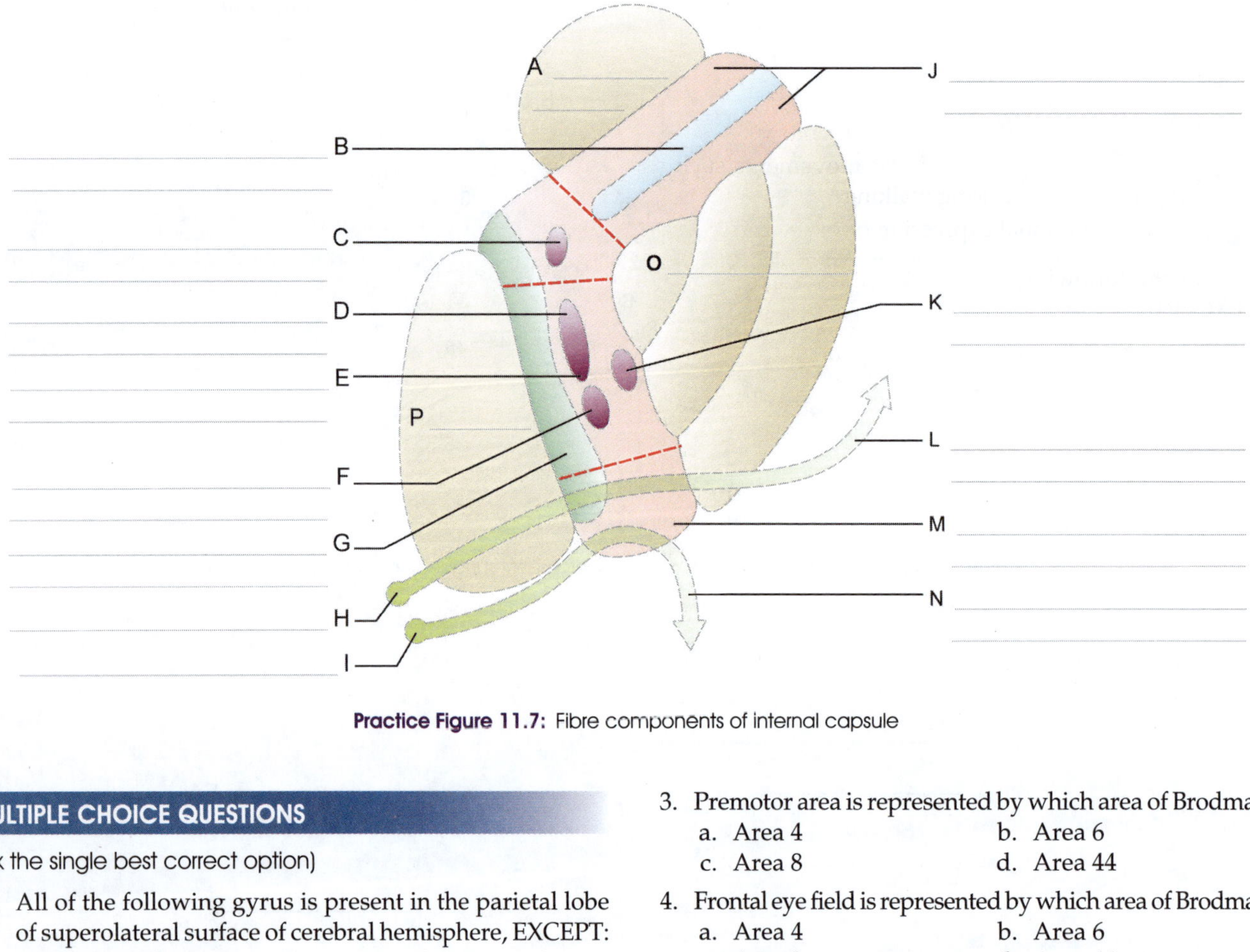


**Practice Figure 11.7:** Fibre components of internal capsule

## MULTIPLE CHOICE QUESTIONS

(Tick the single best correct option)

1. All of the following gyrus is present in the parietal lobe of superolateral surface of cerebral hemisphere, EXCEPT:
   a. Precentral gyrus
   b. Postcentral gyrus
   c. Superior parietal lobule
   d. Inferior parietal lobule
2. Which of the following is not a gyrus on the medial surface of cerebral hemisphere?
   a. Paraterminal  b. Cingulate
   c. Callosal  d. Cuneus
3. Premotor area is represented by which area of Brodmann?
   a. Area 4  b. Area 6
   c. Area 8  d. Area 44
4. Frontal eye field is represented by which area of Brodmann?
   a. Area 4  b. Area 6
   c. Area 8  d. Area 44
5. Motor aphasia is caused due to lesion of which area of Brodmann of cerebral cortex?
   a. Area 4  b. Area 6
   c. Area 8  d. Area 44 and 45
6. Which area of Brodmann is primary visual area?
   a. Area 17  b. Area 18
   c. Area 19  d. Area 22

7. Lesion of which area of cerebral cortex results in astereognosis?
   a. First somesthetic area
   b. Secondary somesthetic area
   c. Sensory association area
   d. Sensory speech area
8. Identify the marked structure with X.

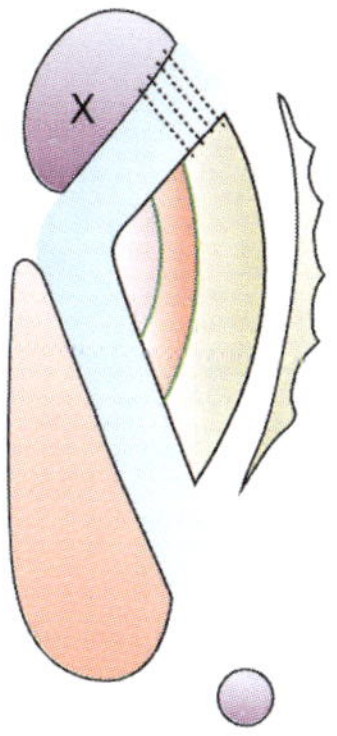


   a. Caudate nucleus   b. Amygdaloid body
   c. Claustrum   d. Internal capsule
9. All of the following is the function of corpus striatum, EXCEPT:
   a. Refinement of reflex and voluntary movements
   b. Learning and retention of recent memory
   c. Controls automatic associated movements such as swinging of arms during walking
   d. Controls emotional expression of movements
10. All of the following is true about amygdaloid body, EXCEPT.
   a. It is a small almond-shaped mass of grey matter in the occipital lobe
   b. It lies anterosuperior to the tip of inferior horn of lateral ventricle
   c. It lies deep to uncus
   d. Functionally, it is related to the limbic system
11. All of the following is symptom of parkinsonism, EXCEPT?
   a. Bradykinesia   b. Stiffness
   c. Hemiballismus   d. Tremors
12. All of the following are projection fibres, EXCEPT:
   a. Corona radiata   b. Internal capsule
   c. Cingulum   d. Fimbria
13. Which of the following are longest association fibres?
   a. Superior longitudinal fasciculus
   b. Inferior longitudinal fasciculus
   c. Uncinate fasciculus
   d. Cingulate fasciculus
14. Which of the following connects motor speech (Broca's) area and orbit gyri of frontal lobe with the cortex of temporal pole?
   a. Superior longitudinal fasciculus
   b. Inferior longitudinal fasciculus
   c. Uncinate fasciculus
   d. Cingulate fasciculus
15. All of the following are commissural fibres, EXCEPT:
   a. Corpus callosum   b. Fornix
   c. Anterior commissure   d. Posterior commissure
16. Which of the following sensory fibres run from medial geniculate body to the primary auditory area of temporal lobe?
   a. Anterior thalamic radiation
   b. Superior thalamic radiation
   c. Inferior thalamic radiation
   d. Posterior thalamic radiation
17. All of the following is true about the lesion of the internal capsule, EXCEPT?
   a. Vascular lesions of the internal capsule are common
   b. It involves rupture of vessels which results in haemorrhage or occlusion
   c. It occurs commonly in the medial and lateral branches of the middle cerebral artery
   d. Lesion of the internal capsule results in lower motor neuron type of paralysis of the opposite half of the body and face

## QUESTION BANK

(Use separate copy to solve the following questions)

Q 1. Describe the sulci and gyri located on the superolateral surface of the cerebrum. Mention the functional areas located on this surface.

Q 2. Describe the internal capsule under the following headings: Features, relations, constituent fibres, blood supply and lesions.

Q 3. Describe the basal ganglia, their connections, and applied aspects.

Q 4. Write a short notes on:
   a. Corpus callosum   b. Broca's area
   c. Sensory aphasia   d. Parkinson's disease.

Chapter

# 12 Lateral Ventricle and Limbic System

eSmartQuiz

## CLINICOANATOMICAL PROBLEM

### Clinical Case 1

A 45-year-old male presented with progressive headaches, nausea, and visual disturbances. Neurological examination revealed papilledema and impaired coordination. MRI of the brain showed significant **dilation of the lateral ventricles**, suggestive of obstructive hydrocephalus. A mass lesion in the region of the third ventricle was identified, indicative of a brain tumour. CSF examination via lumbar puncture revealed elevated protein levels but no signs of infection.

1. Why is the lateral ventricle dilated in this case?
2. Why did the patient have papilledema?

### *Explanation*

1. ______________________________

2. ______________________________

## PRACTICE FIGURES

(Label the practice figures)

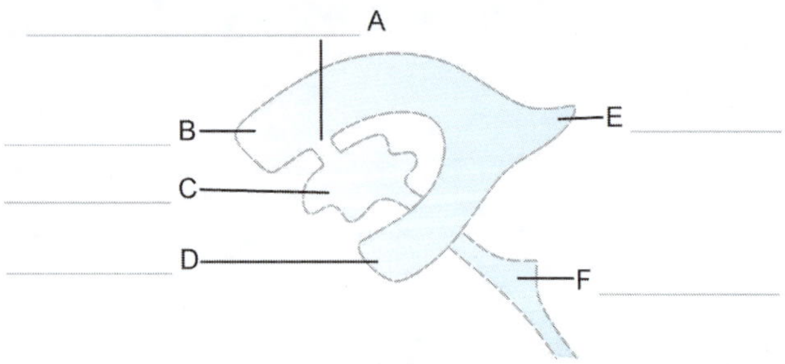


**Practice Figure 12.1:** Ventricles of the brain

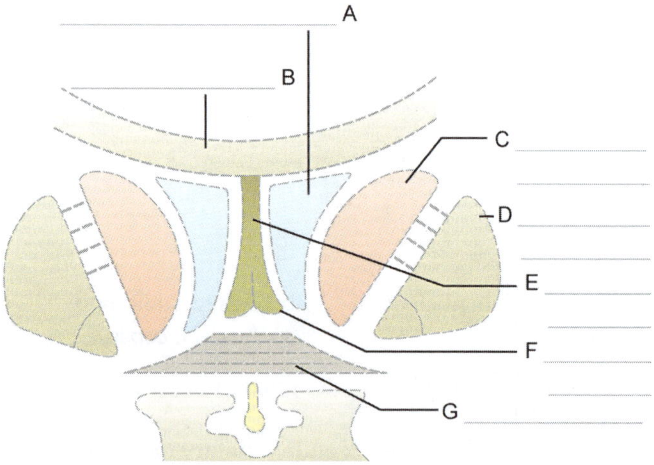


**Practice Figure 12.2:** Anterior horn of lateral ventricle

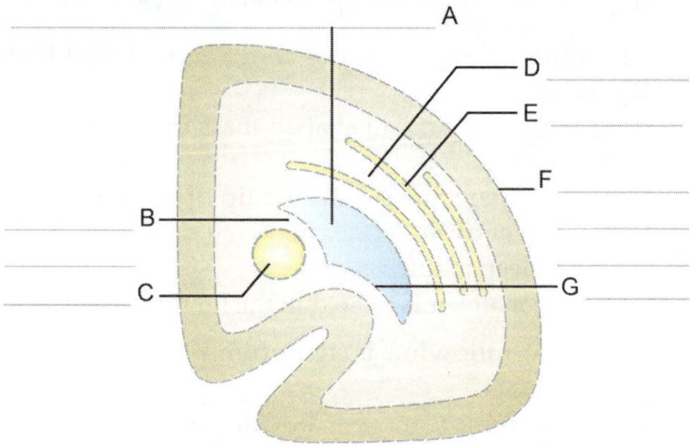


**Practice Figure 12.3:** Posterior horn of lateral ventricle

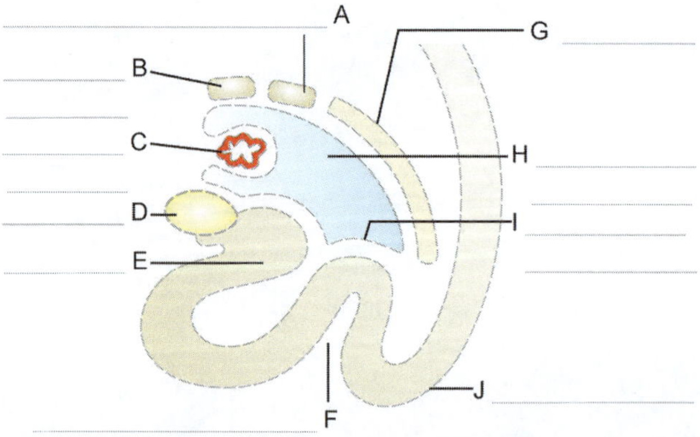


**Practice Figure 12.4:** Inferior horn of lateral ventricle

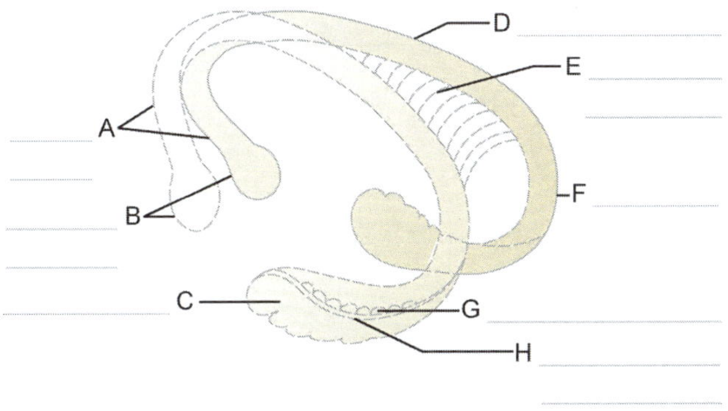


Practice Figure 12.5: Fornix

## MULTIPLE CHOICE QUESTIONS

(Tick the single best correct option)

1. All of the following are parts of hippocampal formation, EXCEPT:
   a. Uncus  b. Hippocampus
   c. Dentate gyrus  d. Indusium griseum
2. All of the following are part of the limbic lobe, EXCEPT:
   a. Paraterminal (subcallosal) gyrus
   b. Cingulate gyrus
   c. Dentate gyrus
   d. Parahippocampal gyrus
3. All of the following are included in primary olfactory area, EXCEPT:
   a. Lateral olfactory gyrus
   b. Hippocampus
   c. Uncus
   d. Gyrus ambiens,
4. Which of the following forms the efferent fibres of amygdaloid body?
   a. Ansa lenticularis  b. Stria terminalis
   c. Lenticular fasciculus  d. Fornix
5. Which of the following is true about Dentate gyrus?
   a. It is a narrow crenated, toothed strip of grey matter
   b. It lies on the upper surface of parahippocampal gyrus
   c. Posteriorly, it is continuous with gyrus fasciolaris through indusium griseum
   d. All of the above
6. Which of the following is an arched bundle of projection fibres from the hippocampus to the mammillary body?
   a. Anterior thalamic radiation
   b. Fornix
   c. Fimbria
   d. Medial longitudinal stria
7. All of the following are components of the Papez circuit, EXCEPT:
   a. Hippocampal formation
   b. Mammillary body
   c. Lateral nucleus of thalamus
   d. Entorhinal cortex
8. Two lateral ventricles are separated from each other by:
   a. Uncus  b. Septum pellucidum
   c. Fornix  d. Indusium griseum
9. Lateral ventricle communicates with the 3rd ventricle through:
   a. Central canal
   b. Foramen of Luschka
   c. Interventricular foramen of Monro
   d. Cerebral aqueduct
10. Which of the following is true about choroid plexus?
    a. It is a highly vascular fold of dura mater
    b. It is a highly vascular fold of arachnoid mater
    c. It is a highly vascular fold of pia mater
    d. It is a highly vascular fold of ependyma
11. Identify the part of the lateral ventricle marked with X.

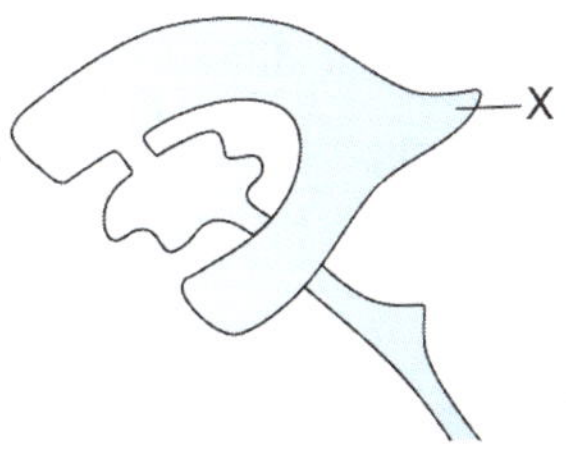


    a. Body  b. Anterior horn
    c. Posterior horn  d. Inferior horn
12. Which of the following do not form the roof of the inferior horn of lateral ventricle?
    a. Tapetum of corpus callosum
    b. Body of caudate nucleus
    c. Stria terminalis
    d. Amygdaloid body

## QUESTION BANK

(Use separate copy to solve the following questions)

Q 1. Describe the lateral ventricle under the following headings: Parts, relations, communications, and applied aspects.

Q 2. Write a short notes on:
   a. Third ventricle
   b. Limbic lobe
   c. Functions of limbic system
   d. Hippocampal formation

Chapter

# 13 Some Neural Pathways and Reticular Formation

eSmartQuiz

## MULTIPLE CHOICE QUESTIONS

(Tick the single best correct option)

1. All of the following are functions of reticular formation, EXCEPT.
   a. It maintains the state of consciousness
   b. It plays an important role in emotion and consolidation of memory
   c. It controls autonomic reflex centres of brainstem
   d. It influences motor activity through extrapyramidal connections
2. The upper motor neuron type of paralysis is characterised by all of the following, EXCEPT:
   a. Loss of the power of voluntary movements
   b. Clasp-knife type of rigidity (hypertonia)
   c. Tendon reflexes are exaggerated
   d. Babinski's sign is negative
3. Lesion of the pyramidal tract causes:
   a. Clasp-knife rigidity
   b. Loss of superficial reflexes
   c. Positive Babinski's sign
   d. All of the above
4. The first order neurons of trigeminothalamic tract are present at:
   a. Trigeminal ganglion
   b. Motor nucleus of trigeminal nerve
   c. Mesencephalic nucleus of trigeminal nerve
   d. Spinal nucleus of trigeminal nerve
5. Proprioceptive fibres from face and head are received by:
   a. Trigeminal ganglion
   b. Motor nucleus of trigeminal nerve
   c. Mesencephalic nucleus of trigeminal nerve
   d. Spinal nucleus of trigeminal nerve
6. Taste sensation is located at:
   a. Precentral gyrus
   b. Paracentral lobule
   c. Postcentral gyrus
   d. Superior parietal lobule
7. Chorda tympani is a branch of __________ cranial nerve.
   a. Fifth
   b. Seventh
   c. Ninth
   d. Eleventh
8. Nucleus tractus solitarious is received fibres from __________ nerve.
   a. Seventh
   b. Ninth
   c. Tenth
   d. All of the above
9. Ascending reticular activating system is formed by:
   a. Great number of collaterals from spinothalamic tract
   b. Trigeminal lemniscus
   c. Auditory pathway
   d. All of these
10. Identify the fibres of the lateral spinothalamic tract marked with X.

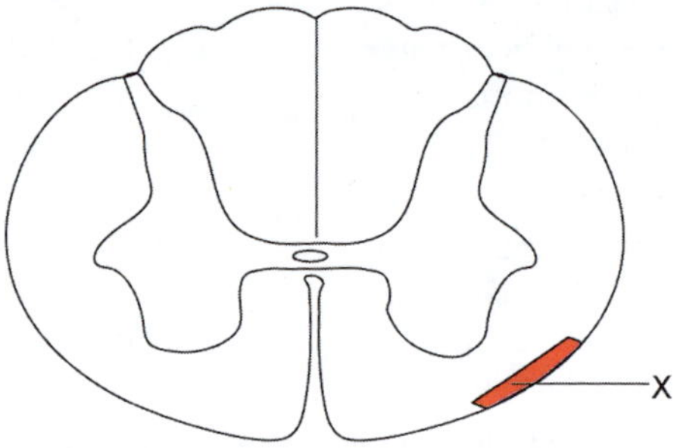


   a. Cervical
   b. Thoracic
   c. Lumbar
   d. Sacral

## QUESTION BANK

(Use separate copy to solve the following question)

Q 1. Write a short notes on:
   a. Reticular formation and connections
   b. Describe the pain pathway.

# Blood Supply of Brain

eSmartQuiz

## CLINICOANATOMICAL PROBLEM

### Clinical Case 1

A 65-year-old male suddenly developed weakness on the right side of his body and difficulty speaking. Neurological examination revealed right-sided hemiplegia and dysarthria. MRI of the brain showed an **infarct in the left internal capsule**, indicative of a vascular lesion.

1. Why did patient have hemiplegia and dysarthria?
2. Which is the artery of cerebral haemorrhage?

*Explanation*

1. ______________________________

2. ______________________________

## PRACTICE FIGURES

(Label the practice figures)

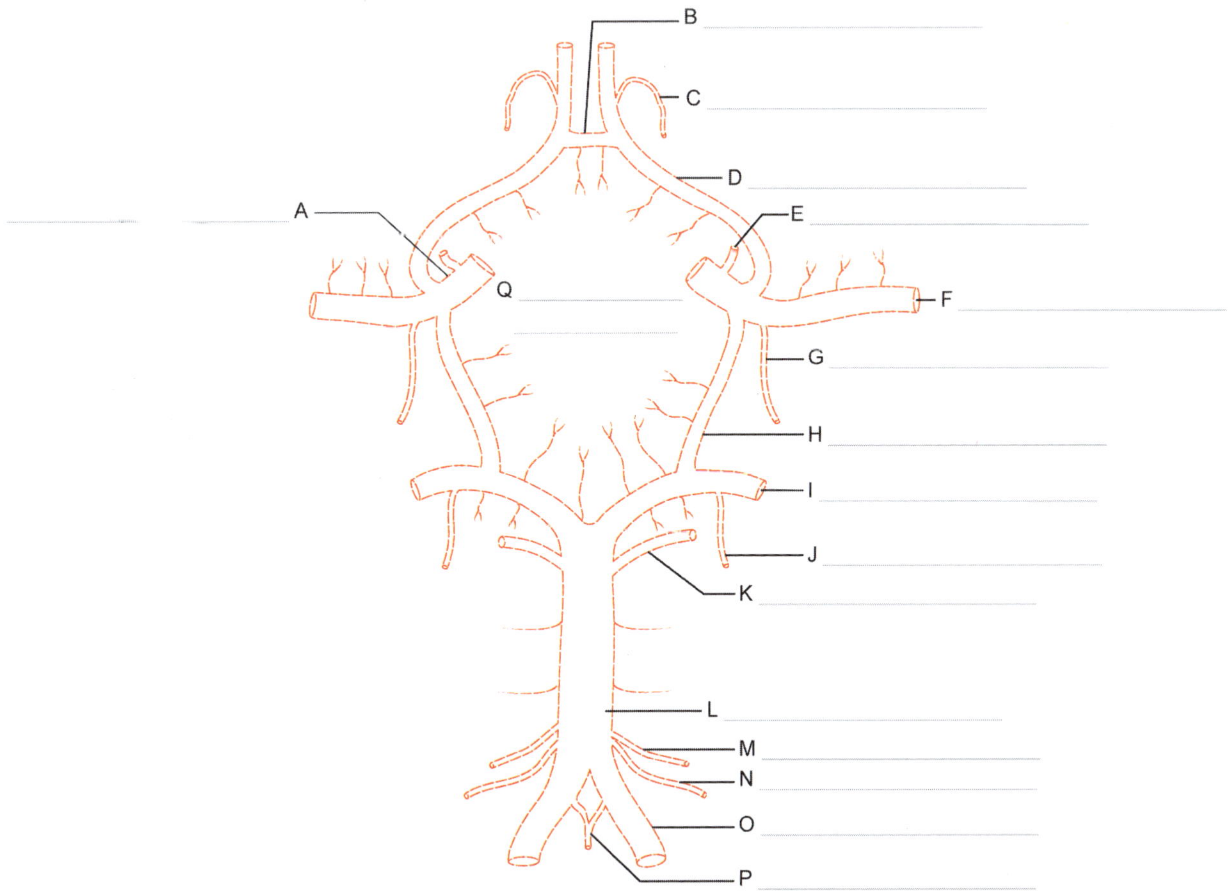


**Practice Figure 14.1:** Circle of Willis

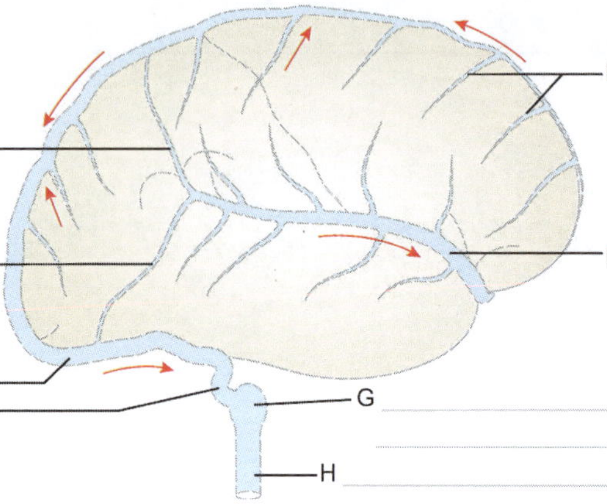


**Practice Figure 14.2:** Veins on the superolateral surface of the cerebral hemisphere (red arrows indicate direction of blood flow)

## MULTIPLE CHOICE QUESTIONS

(Tick the single best correct option)

1. All of the following arteries supply the brain, EXCEPT:
   a. Vertebral artery b. Basilar artery
   c. External carotid artery d. Internal carotid artery
2. Which of the following is the largest branch of 4th part of vertebral artery?
   a. Anterior spinal artery
   b. Posterior spinal artery
   c. Posterior inferior cerebellar artery
   d. Meningeal branch
3. Posterior cerebral arteries are the terminal arteries of:
   a. Vertebral artery b. Basilar artery
   c. External carotid artery d. Internal carotid artery
4. All of the following are the branches of basilar artery, EXCEPT:
   a. Anterior inferior cerebellar artery
   b. Posterior inferior cerebellar artery
   c. Superior cerebellar artery
   d. Posterior cerebral artery
5. Which of the following arteries is the end artery?
   a. Anterior inferior cerebellar artery
   b. Pontine artery
   c. Superior cerebellar artery
   d. Labyrinthine artery
6. Which of the following do not form the circle of Willis?
   a. Anterior cerebral artery
   b. Middle cerebral artery
   c. Posterior cerebral artery
   d. Anterior communicating artery
7. Which of the following are the components of blood–brain barrier?
   a. Capillary endothelium with tight junctions
   b. Basal lamina of endothelium
   c. Processes of astrocytes covering the basal lamina of endothelium
   d. All of the above
8. All of the following areas are devoid of blood–brain barrier, EXCEPT?
   a. Pineal gland b. Corpus callosum
   c. Tuber cinereum d. Choroid plexuses
9. All of the following are the characteristic features of veins of the brain, EXCEPT:
   a. Devoid of muscles b. Devoid of valves
   c. Do follow arteries d. Drain into dural sinuses
10. Which of the following vein lies superficially in the posterior ramus of lateral sulcus and drains into cavernous sinus?
    a. Superior cerebral vein
    b. Superficial middle cerebral vein
    c. Deep middle cerebral vein
    d. Inferior cerebral vein
11. Which of the following vein connects the superficial middle cerebral vein with the transverse sinus?
    a. Superior anastomotic vein of Trolard
    b. Superficial middle cerebral vein
    c. Deep middle cerebral vein
    d. Inferior anastomotic vein of Labbe
12. Basal veins of Rosenthal are formed by the union of all of the following, EXCEPT:
    a. Superficial middle cerebral vein
    b. Deep middle cerebral vein
    c. Anterior cerebral vein
    d. Striate vein
13. Which of the following arteries supply visual fibres?
    a. Anterior and middle cerebral
    b. Middle cerebral and anterior choroidal
    c. Middle and posterior cerebral
    d. Posterior cerebral and anterior cerebral
14. Name the artery supplying the red marked area of the midbrain.

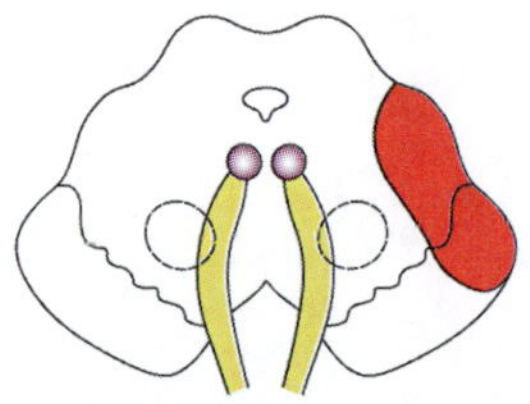

    a. Superior cerebellar artery
    b. Anterior inferior cerebellar artery
    c. Posterior inferior cerebellar artery
    d. Anterior cerebral artery

## QUESTION BANK

(Use separate copy to solve the following question)

Q 1. Write a short notes on:
   a. Circle of Willis
   b. Blood–brain barrier
   c. Great cerebral vein of Galen
   d. Blood supply of spinal cord

Chapter 15

# Surface Marking and Radiological Anatomy of Nervous System

eSmartQuiz

## PRACTICE FIGURE

(Label the practice figure)

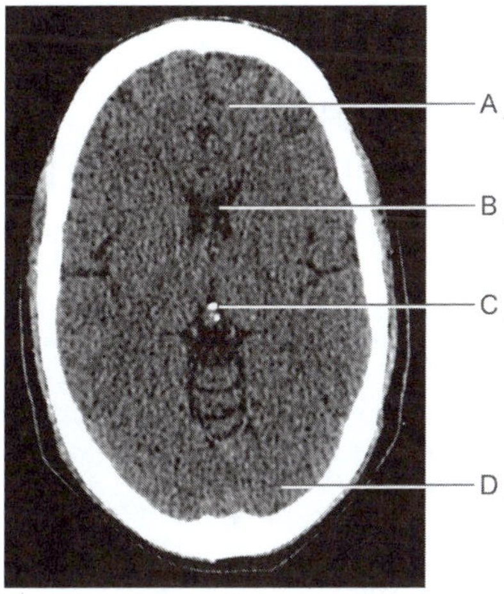


**Practice Figure 15.1:** Calcified pineal gland (due to aging) on CT scan

## MULTIPLE CHOICE QUESTIONS

(Tick the single best correct option)

1. Identify the following image.
   a. Plain radiograph
   b. CT scan
   c. MRI
   d. PET scan

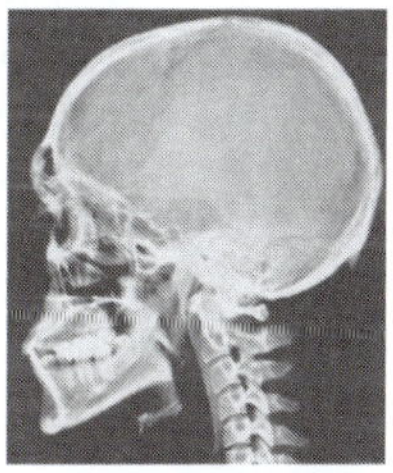

2. Identify the following image.
   a. Plain radiograph
   b. CT scan
   c. MRI
   d. PET scan

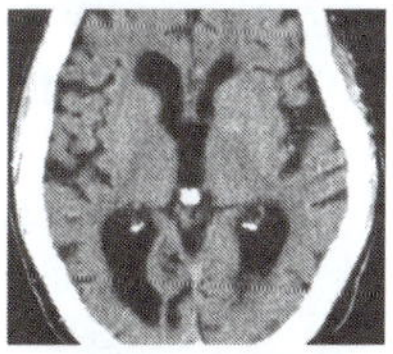

3. Identify the following image.
   a. Plain radiograph
   b. CT scan
   c. MRI
   d. PET scan

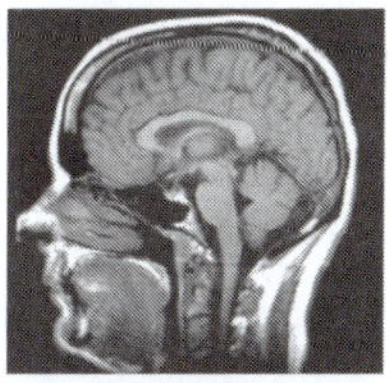

4. Identify the following image.
   a. Plain radiograph
   b. CT scan
   c. MRI
   d. PET scan

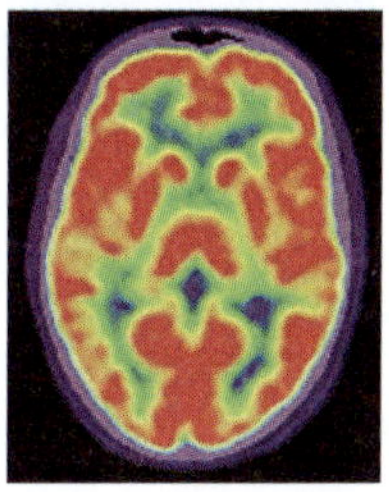

5. Identify the following image.

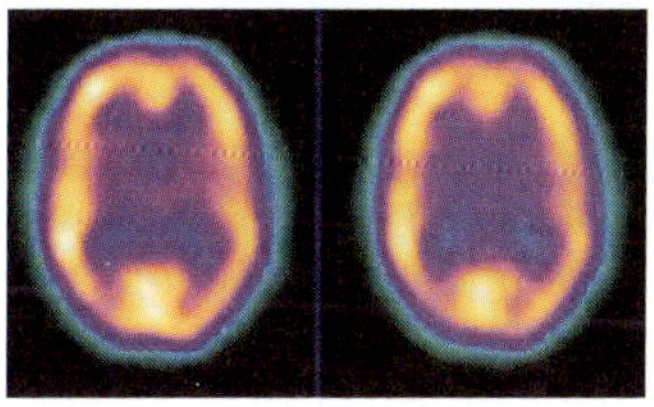

   a. MRI  b. PET scan
   c. SPECT scan  d. Contrast CT scan

6. Identify the structure marked with X.

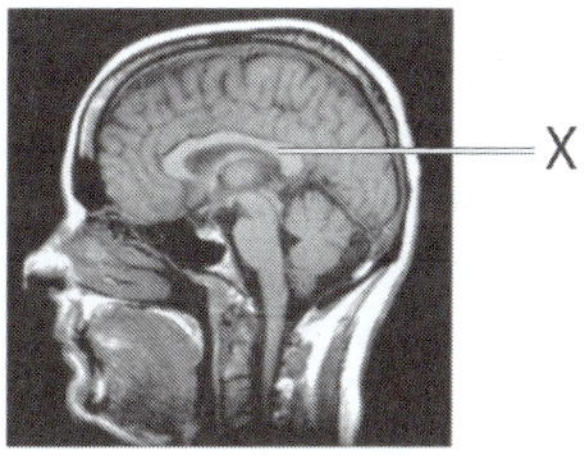


   a. Cerebellum  b. Cingulate gyrus
   c. Pons  d. Corpus callosum

7. Identify the part of the lateral ventricle marked with X.

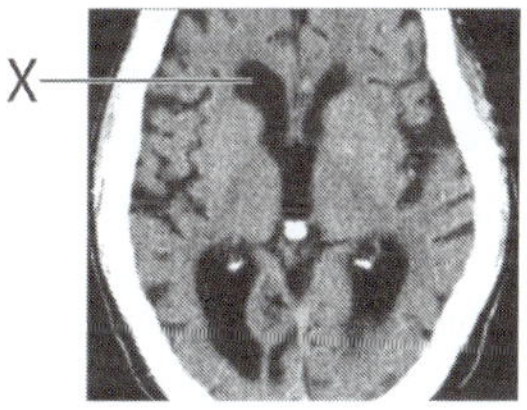


   a. Anterior horn  b. Posterior horn
   c. Body  d. Inferior horn

8. Gamma-ray-emitting radioisotopes are useful for:
   a. Cerebral angiography
   b. PET scan
   c. SPECT scan
   d. Contrast CT scan

9. The metabolic activity of the brain is detected by using:
   a. Cerebral angiography
   b. PET scan
   c. SPECT scan
   d. Contrast CT scan

10. Pyelocil dye is useful for:
    a. Cerebral angiography
    b. PET scan
    c. SPECT scan
    d. Contrast CT scan

Chapter

# 16

eSmartQuiz

# Autonomic Nervous System

## CLINICOANATOMICAL PROBLEM

### Clinical Case 1

A 6-month-old male infant presented with chronic constipation and abdominal distension since birth. Physical examination revealed a palpable mass in the abdomen. Imaging studies showed dilated loops of the colon. Further evaluation with rectal biopsy confirmed the diagnosis of **congenital megacolon**.

1. What is another name for congenital megacolon?
2. What is structure absent in colon in this disease?

### *Explanation*

1. ______________________________

______________________________

2. ______________________________

______________________________

## MULTIPLE CHOICE QUESTIONS

(Tick the single best correct option)

1. All the following statements are true about the sympathetic nervous system, EXCEPT:
   a. It is called the thoracolumbar system or outflow
   b. The parasympathetic ganglia are located near the viscera
   c. Postganglionic fibres are non-myelinated
   d. Postganglionic fibre neurotransmitters are adrenaline, noradrenaline and acetylcholine
2. All the following statements are true about the parasympathetic nervous system, EXCEPT:
   a. It is called the craniosacral system or outflow
   b. The parasympathetic ganglia are located near the viscera
   c. Postganglionic fibres are long and non-myelinated
   d. Postganglionic fibre neurotransmitter is acetylcholine
3. All the following are the functions of the parasympathetic nervous system, EXCEPT:
   a. Decreases heart rate, force of contraction, and cardiac output
   b. Decreases respiratory rate
   c. Bronchoconstriction
   d. Vasoconstriction in the skin and gut
4. All the following are the functions of the sympathetic nervous system, EXCEPT:
   a. Increases heart rate, force of contraction, and cardiac output
   b. Increases respiratory rate
   c. Bronchoconstriction
   d. Vasoconstriction in the skin and gut
5. All the following are the functions of the sympathetic nervous system, EXCEPT:
   a. Peristalsis – decreases
   b. Sphincters – contract
   c. Secretions – decrease
   d. Pupil – constriction
6. All the following are the functions of the parasympathetic nervous system, EXCEPT:
   a. Peristalsis – increases
   b. Sphincters – contract
   c. Secretions – increase
   d. Pupil – constriction
7. All the following are the parasympathetic ganglia, EXCEPT:
   a. Ciliary ganglion
   b. Coeliac ganglion
   c. Otic ganglion
   d. Submandibular ganglion
8. All the following are the sympathetic ganglia, EXCEPT:
   a. Ciliary ganglion
   b. Coeliac ganglion
   c. Superior mesenteric ganglion
   d. Inferior mesenteric ganglion
9. Sacral outflow of the parasympathetic system include:
   a. Only S1 and S2 segments
   b. Only S2 and S3 segments
   c. S2, S3, and S2 segments
   d. S3, S4, and S5 segments
10. Which of the following cranial nerve does not carry parasympathetic fibres?
    a. Third   b. Fourth
    c. Seventh   d. Eighth

## QUESTION BANK

(Use separate copy to solve the following question)

Q 1. List the differences between sympathetic and autonomic nervous systems.

Chapter

17

# Development of Nervous System

eSmartQuiz

## CLINICOANATOMICAL PROBLEM

### Clinical Case 1

A 32-year-old female presented with chronic lower back pain exacerbated by prolonged sitting and standing. Physical examination revealed no obvious spinal deformities but highlighted tenderness over the lower lumbar vertebrae. Imaging, including MRI, revealed a bony defect in the vertebral arches consistent with **spina bifida occulta**.

1. What is spina bifida occulta?
2. What is the embryological basis for spina bifida?
3. What are other types of spina bifida?

### *Explanation*

1. ______________________________

2. ______________________________

3. ______________________________

## MULTIPLE CHOICE QUESTIONS

(Tick the single best correct option)

1. What is the remnant of anterior neuropore in later life?
   a. Lamina terminalis  b. Terminal ventricle
   c. Pineal body  d. Cerebral aqueduct
2. Which of the following is developed from diencephalon?
   a. Hypothalamus  b. Midbrain
   c. Cerebellum  d. Medulla oblongata
3. All are the neural derivatives of neural crest cells, EXCEPT:
   a. Satellite cell in ganglion
   b. Schwann cells
   c. Dorsal root ganglia
   d. Microglia
4. What is the embryonic source of microglial cells?
   a. Neural crest cells  b. Mesenchymal tissues
   c. Pluripotent cells  d. Spongioblast cells
5. All are the derivatives of neural crest cells, EXCEPT:
   a. Odontoblast of teeth
   b. Parafollicular cells of thyroid gland
   c. Glomus (type I) cells
   d. Glomus (type II) cells
6. All of the following statements is true, EXCEPT:
   a. Neuroblasts form purkinje cells of cerebellum
   b. Oligodendroglial cells develop from glioblasts
   c. Myelination is complete by birth
   d. Parafollicular cells of thyroid gland are derived from neural crest cells

## PRACTICE FIGURE

(Label the practice figure)

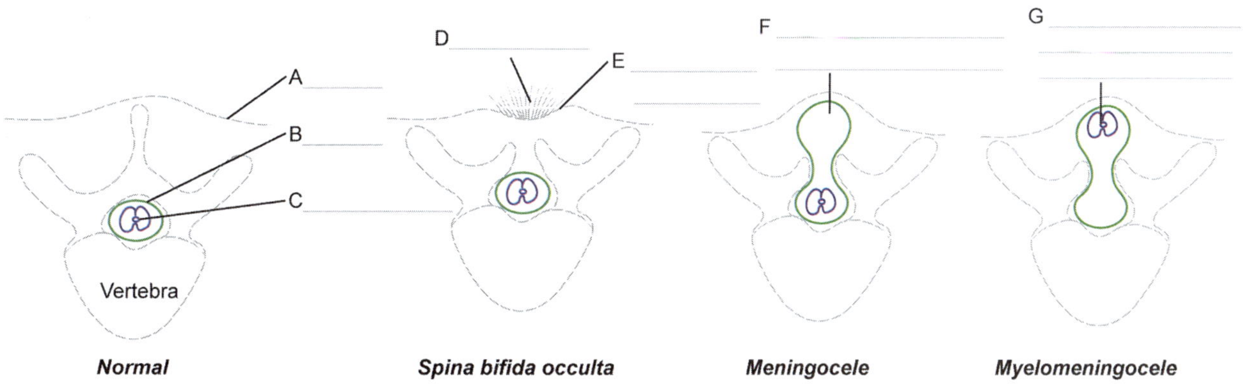


**Practice Figure 17.1:** Types of spina bifida

7. At birth, lower end of spinal cord is located at what level of vertebra?
   a. L1  b. L2
   c. L3  d. L4
8. Which of the following is the derivative of neural crest cells?
   a. Pia mater
   b. Arachnoid mater
   c. Dura mater
   d. None of the above
9. All of the following statements are true about myelination, EXCEPT:
   a. Myelination begins when the nerve fibres start functioning
   b. It begins during the 4th month of IUL and continues after the birth up to 2–3 years
   c. Sensory fibres myelinate earlier than motor fibres
   d. Myelination in the central nervous system is the function of oligodendrocytes
10. Myelination in peripheral nervous system is the function of ____________.
    a. Oligodendrocytes  b. Schwann cells
    c. Microglial cells  d. Ependymal cells
11. Myelination in central nervous system is the function of ____________.
    a. Oligodendrocytes  b. Schwann cells
    c. Microglial cells  d. Ependymal cells
12. What is the condition in which there is enlargement of central canal of spinal cord?
    a. Anencephaly  b. Encephalocele
    c. Syringomyelia  d. Meningocele
13. A 30-year-old pregnant woman at 18 weeks of gestation comes to the physician for a normal examination. During routine blood tests, her serum alpha-fetoprotein (AFP) concentration is found to be markedly decreased for her gestational age. Which abnormality will the physician need to rule out based on these low AFP levels?
    a. Spina bifida  b. Anencephaly
    c. Meningocele  d. Down syndrome

## QUESTION BANK

(Use separate copy to solve the following question)

Q 1. Write a short notes on:
   a. Spina bifida
   b. Positional changes of spinal cord with the age

# Spotters in Head and Neck and Brain–Neuroanatomy

## Answer the Questions for the given Spotters or Objective Structured Practical Examination (OSPE).

*Note*: The purpose of the spotters given here is to orient the students for the practical examination pattern. However, numerous other questions may come for spotters as well. For bone, side determination is important. For muscles, nerve supply and actions are important. For arteries and nerves, their branches are important for spotter examination.

### Spotter 1

a. Name the structures attached to the part of the bone marked green.

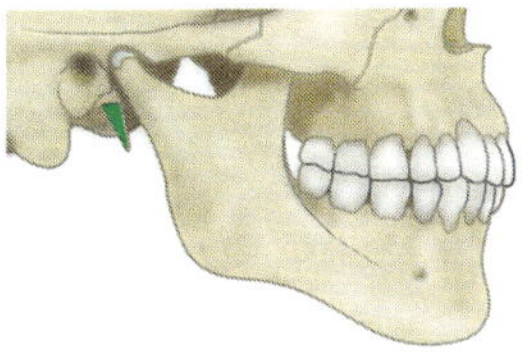

(*Other possible spotters*: Relations of pterion, bregma, attachment of zygomatic arch, masseter, temporalis, medial and lateral pterygoid and various foramina)

### Spotter 2

a. Identify the vertebra.
b. Name the structures passing through the foramina located on its transverse process.

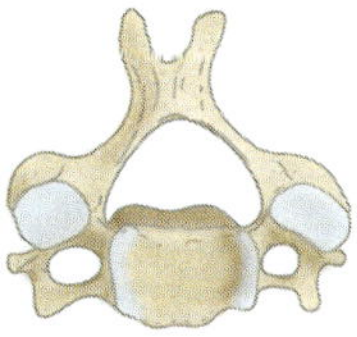

(*Other possible spotters*: Identification feature, carotid tubercle, joints formed and their types. Atlas vertebra – identification, Axis vertebra – identification, attachments of dens)

### Spotter 3

a. Name the structure marked with X.
b. Name its branches.

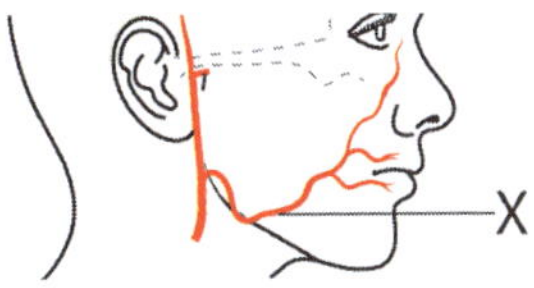


(*Other possible spotters*: External carotid artery and its branches, common carotid artery and its level of bifurcation)

### Spotter 4

a. Name the structure marked with X.
b. Write its nerve supply.

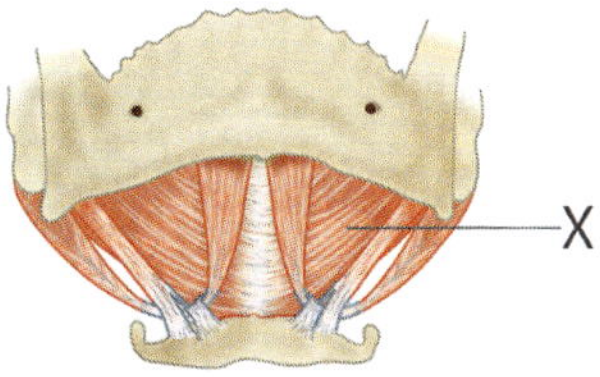


(*Other possible spotters*: Digastric, temporalis, masseter, medial and lateral pterygoid muscles– Identification, nerve supply, actions)

### Spotter 5

a. Identify the muscle marked with X.
b. What is its nerve supply?

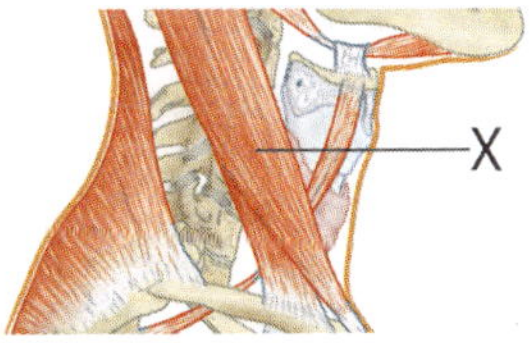


(*Other possible spotters*: Actions, trapezius, muscles in the floor of the posterior triangle, muscles of the anterior triangle)

### Spotter 6

a. Name the structure marked with X.
b. Name any one muscle supplied by it.

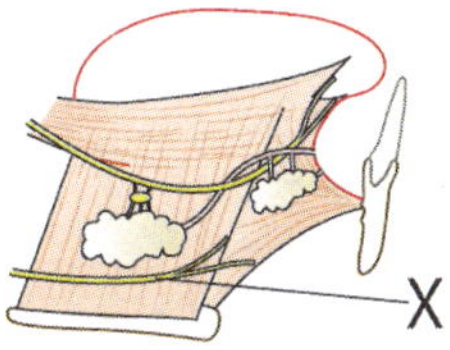

## Spotter 7

a. Name the structure marked with X.
b. Name the arteries supplying it.

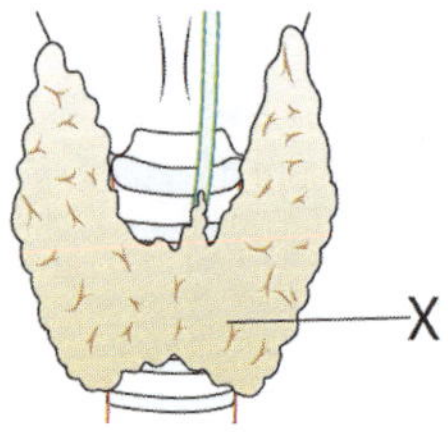


(*Other possible spotters*: Thyroid gland: Capsules, hormones secreted. Parotid gland: identification, duct, intraglandular structures. Submandibular gland: identification, parts, relations, duct)

## Spotter 8

a. Identify the nerve.
b. Name any two muscles supplied by it.

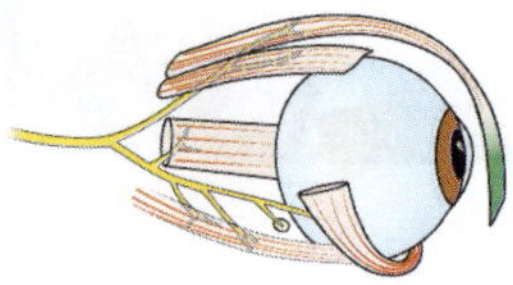

(*Other possible spotters*: Actions of extraocular muscles, trochlear nerve, frontal nerve, ophthalmic artery)

## Spotter 9

a. Name the structure marked with X.
b. What type of cartilage is present in it.

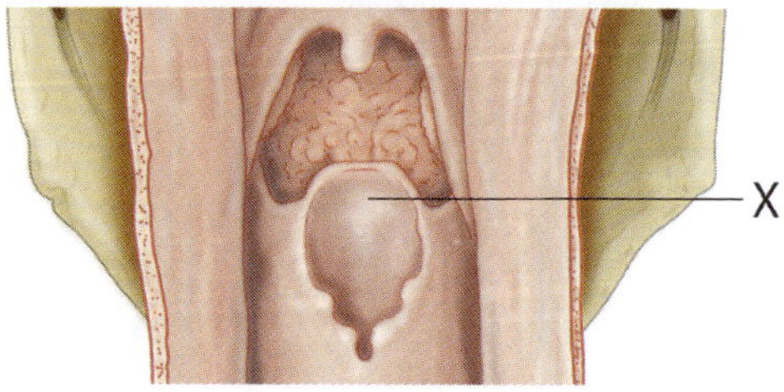


(*Other possible spotters*: Piriform fossa, vallecula, soft palate, laryngeal inlet, vocal cords)

## Spotter 10

a. Name the area marked red.
b. Name the openings in it.

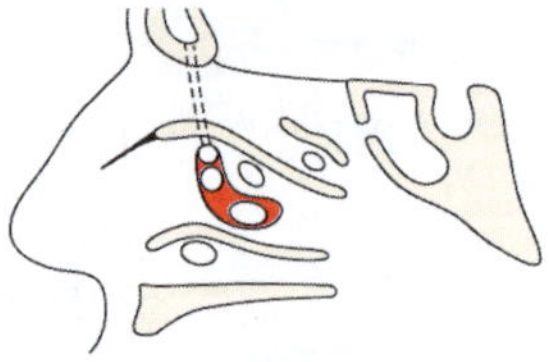

(*Other possible spotters*: Nasal septum – blood supply, nerve supply. Lateral wall of nose: blood supply, nerve supply. Opening of auditory tube and its function)

## Spotter 11

a. Name the structure marked with X.
b. What type of cartilage is it?

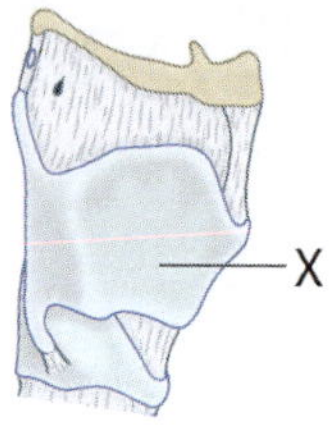


(*Other possible spotters*: Cricoid cartilage, lateral cricothyroid muscle and its functions)

## Spotter 12

a. Name the structure marked with X.
b. What is its nerve supply.

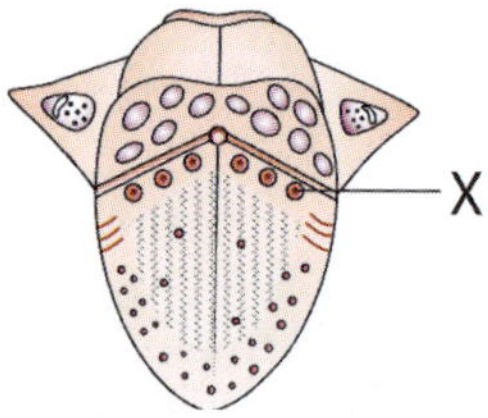


(*Other possible spotters*: Nerve supply of tongue, development of tongue and its applied aspects)

## Spotter 13

a. Name the structure marked with X.
b. Where does this sinus opens?

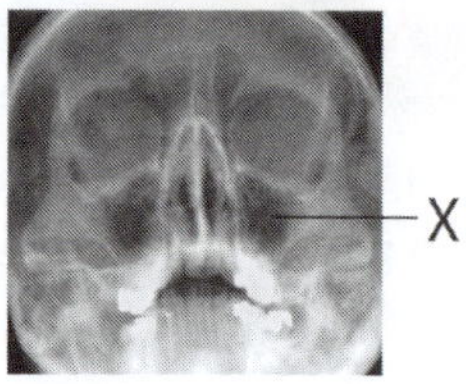


(*Other possible spotters*: Frontal air sinus, ethmoidal air sinus, sella turcica)

## Spotter 14

a. Name the structure marked with X.
b. What happens in its lesion?

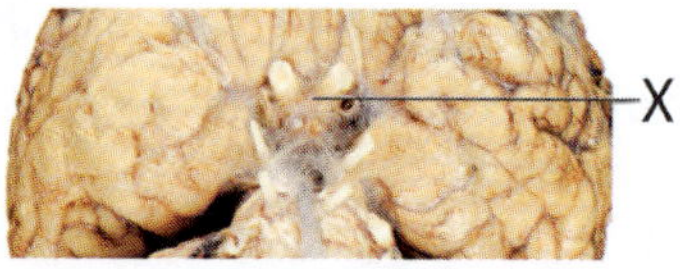


(*Other possible spotters*: Visual pathway, pituitary gland, circle of Willis, olfactory bulb and tract)

## Spotter 15

a. Name the structure marked with X.
b. Write its parts.

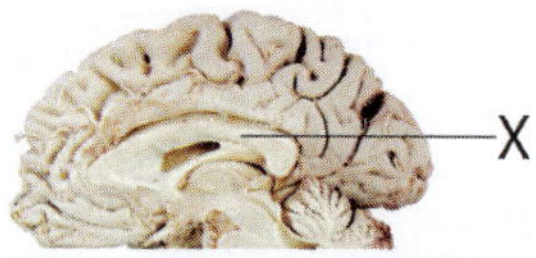


(*Other possible spotters*: Functions, type of fibres, other commissural fibres of cerebrum, fornix, septum pellucidum, interventricular foramen)

## Spotter 16

a. Name the structure marked with X.
b. Name the cranial nerve nuclei present at this level.

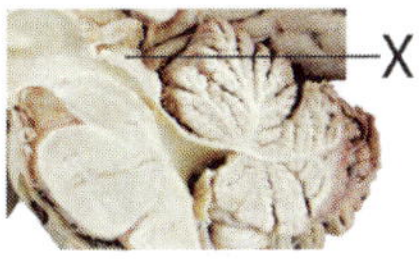


(*Other possible spotters*: Midbrain – inferior colliculus, pons, medulla, 4th ventricle, cerebellum)

## Spotter 17

a. Name the structure marked with X.
b. Write its lateral relations.

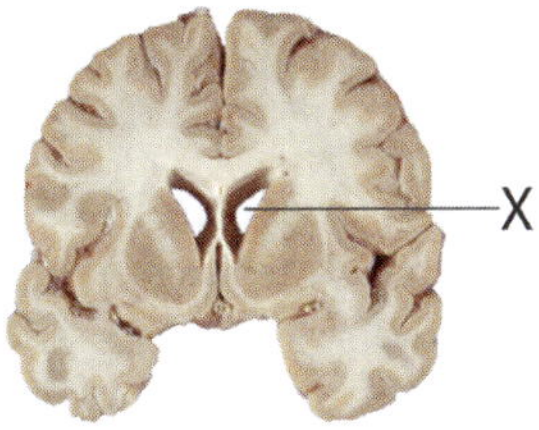


(*Other possible spotters*: Internal capsule, caudate nucleus, corpus callosum)

## Spotter 18

a. Name the structure marked with X.
b. Which cranial nerve nucleus lies deep to it?

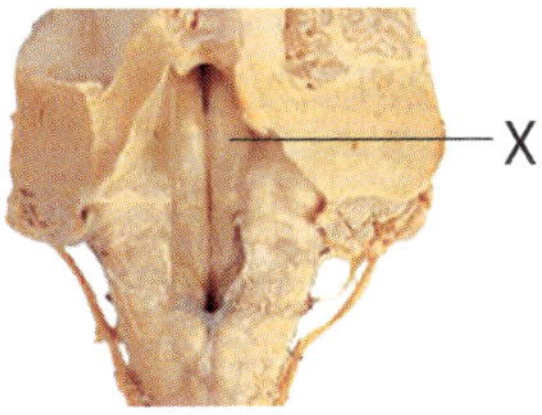


(*Other possible spotters*: Middle cerebral peduncle, vagal triangle, midbrain colliculi)

## Spotter 19

a. Identify the marked cavity.
b. What will happen if it gets blocked?

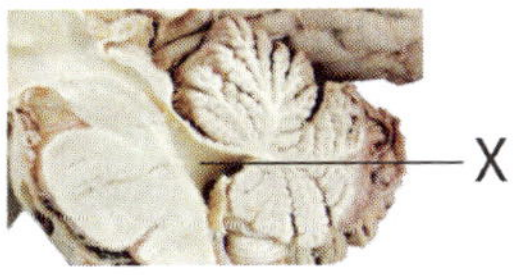


(*Other possible spotters*: Cerebral aqueduct, parts of cerebellum, pons, medulla)

## Spotter 20

a. Name the structure marked with X.
b. Name the Brodmann area located in it.

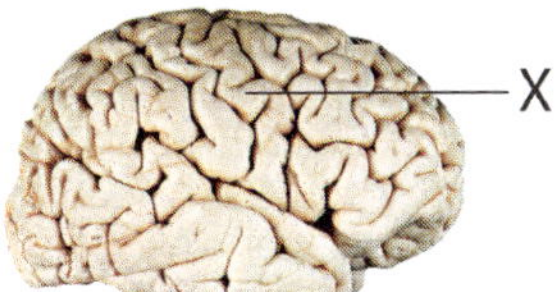


(*Other possible spotters*: Central sulcus, lateral sulcus, postcentral gyrus, visual area, Broca's area)

## Spotter 21

a. Name the structure marked with X.
b. Name its branches.

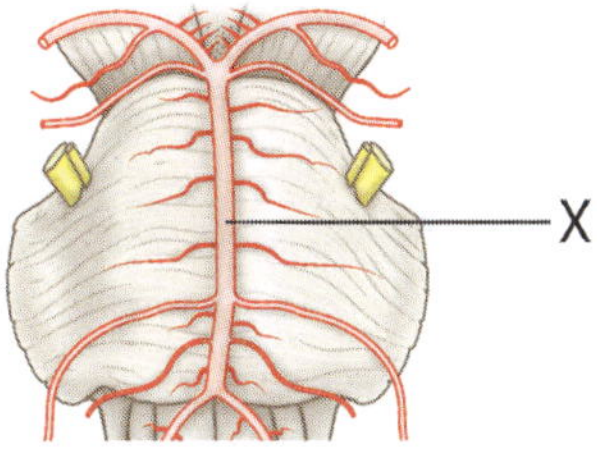


(*Other possible spotters*: Vertebral artery, posterior cerebral artery)

## Spotter 22

a. Name the radiological method used in the following figure.
b. Identify the X-marked part of the brain.

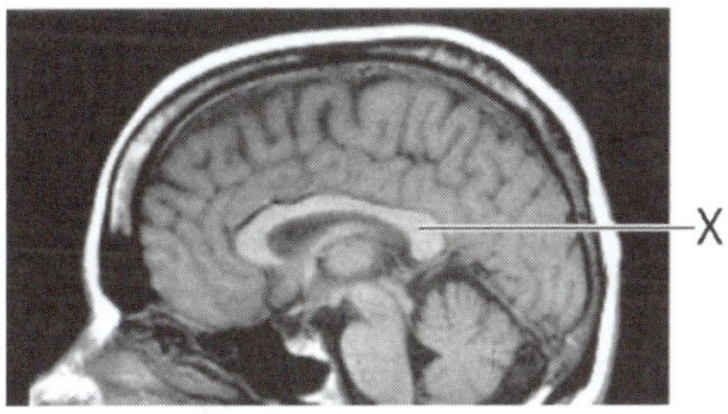


(*Other possible spotters*: Ventricles of brain)

## Spotter 23

a. Name the radiological method used in the following figure.
b. Name the structure marked with X.

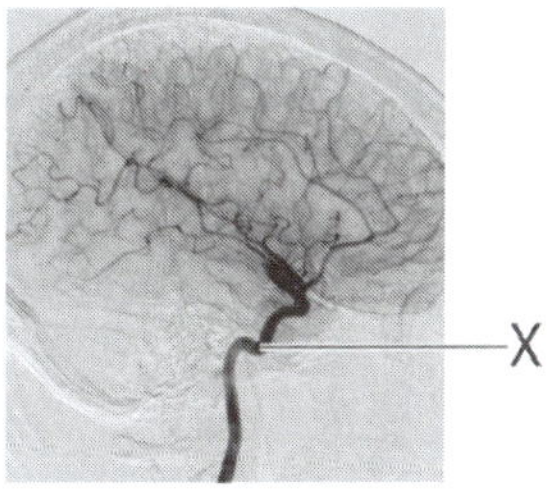


(*Other possible spotters*: Other branches of vertebral artery, circle of Willis, Internal carotid artery)

## Spotter 24

a. Name the structure marked with X.
b. Write its parts.

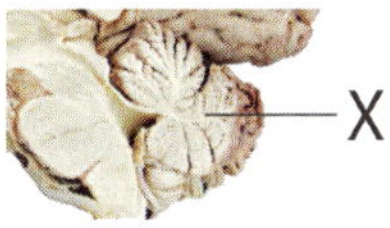


(*Other possible spotters*: Functions of cerebellum)

## Spotter 25

a. Name the structure marked with X.
b. Write its parts.

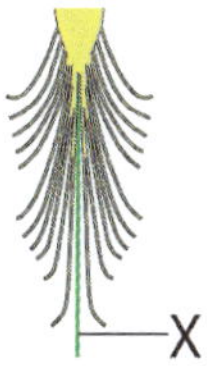


(*Other possible spotters*: Conus medullaris, ligamentum dentaticulum)

Scan to get key

# Answers

## HEAD AND NECK

### Chapter 1

#### Key to Clinicoanatomical Problems

**Clinical Case 1**

1. The pterion is a region on the lateral aspect of the skull where the frontal, parietal, temporal and sphenoid bones converge.
2. Middle meningeal artery.

**Clinical Case 2**

1. The anterior fontanelle is a diamond-shaped gap at the junction of the coronal and sagittal sutures in the newborn's skull.
2. Between 12 to 18 months of age.
3. Posterior fontanelle, mastoid (posterolateral) fontanelles, sphenoid (anterolateral) fontanelles.

#### Key to Practice Figures

**Practice Figure 1.1**

A. Supraorbital notch, B. Nasal bone, C. Infraorbital foramen, D. Mental foramen, E. Frontal bone, F. Superciliary arch, G. Orbital opening, H. Zygomatic bone, I. Anterior nasal aperture, J. Maxilla, K. Mandible

**Practice Figure 1.2**

A. Parietal bone, B. Superior temporal line, C. Inferior temporal line, D. Temporal bone, E. Lambdoid suture, F. Occipital bone, G. Asterion, H. External auditory meatus, I. Mastoid process, J. Styloid process, K. Coronal suture, L. Frontal bone, M. Pterion, N. Greater wing of sphenoid, O. Nasal bone, P. Zygomatic arch, Q. Zygomatic bone, R. Maxilla, S. Mandible

**Practice Figure 1.3**

A. Posterior fontanelle, B. Occipital bone, C. Mastoid (posterolateral) fontanelle, D. Anterior fontanelle, E. Frontal bone, F. Sphenoidal (anterolateral) fontanelle, G. Maxilla, H. Mandible, I. Parietal bone

**Practice Figure 1.4**

A. Masseter, B. Temporalis, C. Buccinator, D. Depressor anguli oris, E. Depressor labii inferioris, F. Mentalis, G. Platysma, H. Lateral pterygoid, I. Temporalis, J. Pterygomandibular raphe, K. Genioglossus, L. Geniohyoid, M. Anterior belly of digastric, N. Superior constrictor, O. Medial pterygoid, P. Mylohyoid

**Practice Figure 1.5**

A. Stylohyoid ligament, B. Genioglossus, C. Geniohyoid, D. Mylohyoid, E. Sternohyoid, F. Middle constrictor, G. Hyoglossus, H. Thyrohyoid, I. Stylohyoid (2 slips), J. Omohyoid (superior belly)

**Practice Figure 1.6**

A. Bifid spine, B. Lamina, C. Superior articular facet, D. Posterior root, E. Posterior tubercle, F. Costotransverse bar, G. Foramen transversarium, H. Anterior root, I. Anterior tubercle, J. Vertebral foramen, K. Body

**Practice Figure 1.7**

A. Vertebral artery, B. Rectus capitis posterior minor, C. Obliquus superior, D. Levator scapulae, E. Rectus capitis lateralis, F. Rectus capitis anterior, G. Odontoid process, H. Transverse ligament, I. C1 nerve

#### Key to MCQs

1. a 2. c 3. d 4. c 5. b 6. c 7. a
8. b 9. b 10. d 11. b 12. c 13. b

### Chapter 2

#### Key to Clinicoanatomical Problems

**Clinical Case 1**

1. Stylomastoid foramen.
2. a. Orbicularis oculi muscle
   b. Orbicularis oris muscle.

**Clinical Case 2**

1. The eye turned black due to extension of the blood from the scalp to the upper eyelid thorough the loose connective tissue layer of the scalp. The accumulation of blood in the tissues around the eye, known as periorbital hematoma.
2. Because the scalp has a rich supply of blood vessels.

**Clinical Case 3**

1. The central region of the face, including the nose, upper lip, and cheeks. Its infections easily spread to the intracranial structures due to the venous connections.
2. The infection from the upper lip spread to the meninges through the facial veins, which communicate with the cavernous sinus via the deep facial veins. The lack of valves in these veins allows retrograde spread of infection.

**Clinical Case 4**

1. It is a case of cephalohematoma.
2. The selling is due to a subperiosteal collection of blood between the skull bone and its periosteum, caused by the vacuum assistance during delivery.
3. It is usually located on one side of the head. It typically does not cross suture lines because the periosteum does not extend across them.

#### Key to Practice Figures

**Practice Figure 2.1**

A. Skin, B. Connective tissue, C. Aponeurotic layer, D. Loose areolar tissue, E. Pericranium, F. Superior sagittal sinus, G. Falx cerebri, H. Emissary vein

**Practice Figure 2.2**

A. Supratrochlear artery, B. Supraorbital artery, C. Superficial temporal artery, D. Posterior auricular artery, E. Occipital artery, F. Supratrochlear nerve, G. Supraorbital nerve, H. Zygomaticotemporal nerve, I. Temporal branch of facial nerve, J. Auriculotemporal nerve, K. Posterior auricular nerve, L. Great auricular nerve, M. Lesser occipital nerve, N. Greater occipital nerve, O. Third occipital nerve

**Practice Figure 2.3**

A. Auricularis anterior, B. Auricularis superior, C. Auricularis posterior, D. Occipitalis, E. Buccinator, F. Risorius, G. Platysma, S. Mentalis, H. Frontalis, I. Corrugator supercilia, J. Procerus, K. Orbicularis oculi, L. Levator labii superioris alaeque nasi, M. Compressor naris, N. Dilator nares, O. Depressor septi, P. Orbicularis oris, Q. Depressor anguli oris, R. Depressor labii inferioris

**Practice Figure 2.4**

A. Orbital part of lacrimal gland, B. Palpebral part of lacrimal gland, C. Lacrimal ducts, D. Conjunctival sac, E. Levator palpebrae superioris, F. Lacrimal punctum, G. Lacrimal canaliculus, H. Lacrimal sac, I. Nasolacrimal duct, J. Inferior meatus of nose, K. Lacrimal fold (valve of Hasner)

#### Key to MCQs

1. c 2. b 3. d 4. b 5. c 6. a 7. c
8. b 9. c 10. b 11. c

## Chapter 3

### Key to Clinicoanatomical Problem

#### *Clinical Case 1*

1. Spinal accessory nerve.
2. Due to paralysis of the trapezius muscle.
3. Damage to the spinal accessory nerve in the posterior triangle of the neck. Before the entry of the spinal accessory nerve in the posterior triangle, it supply sternocleidomastoid muscle.

### Key to Practice Figures

**Practice Figure 3.1**

A. Carotid sheath, B. External carotid artery, C. Internal carotid artery, D. Vagus nerve, E. Internal jugular vein, F. Common carotid artery

**Practice Figure 3.2**

A. Lesser occipital nerve, B. Great auricular nerve, C. Supraclavicular nerves, D. Anterior cutaneous nerve, E. External jugular vein draining into subclavian vein

**Practice Figure 3.3**

A. Muscles forming the floor, B. Semispinalis capitis, C. Splenius capitis, D. Levator scapulae, E. Scalenus medius, F. Sternocleidomastoid, G. Trapezius, H. Clavicle

**Practice Figure 3.4**

A. Splenius capitis muscle, B. Spinal accessory nerve, C. Branches (C3, C4) to trapezius, D. Nerve to serratus anterior, E. Suprascapular nerve, F. Trunks of brachial plexus, G. Lesser occipital nerve, H. Great auricular nerve, I. Anterior (transverse) cutaneous nerve, J. Supraclavicular nerve, K. Nerve to rhomboids, L. Scalenus anterior with phrenic nerve, M. Subclavian vein, N. Nerve to subclavius

### Key to MCQs

1. a  2. d  3. a  4. c  5. a  6. b  7. d
8. b  9. c  10. d

## Chapter 4

### Key to Clinicoanatomical Problems

#### *Clinical Case 1*

1. The carotid sinus is a dilated part in the terminal part of common carotid artery. It contains baroreceptors that help regulate blood pressure.
2. During shaving, the simulation of the carotid sinus due to applied pressure, triggered a sudden drop in heart rate and blood pressure, causing fainting (syncope).
3. Periarterial neurectomy is a surgical procedure involving the removal of the nerve fibres around an artery.
4. This surgery targets the nerve fibres around the carotid sinus to reduce its hypersensitivity, preventing the abnormal reflex that leads to syncope.

#### *Clinical Case 2*

1. Common carotid artery at the anterior border of the sternocleido-mastoid muscle.
2. Superficial temporal and facial arteries.
3. Radial artery.

#### *Clinical Case 3*

1. External jugular vein and subclavian vein.
2. Condition where air bubbles enter the bloodstream, which can obstruct blood flow, leading to respiratory distress, cardiovascular collapse, and potentially death.
3. Reasons: The veins have thin walls and less smooth muscle and it is attached to the surrounding deep fascia.

### Key to Practice Figures

**Practice Figure 4.1**

A. Submental lymph nodes, B. Mylohyoid muscle, C. Median raphe, D. Anterior belly of digastric muscle, E. Hyoid bone, F. Anterior jugular vein

**Practice Figure 4.2**

A. Styloid process, B. Glossopharyngeal nerve, C. Hypoglossal nerve, D. Internal jugular vein, E. Internal carotid artery, F. External carotid artery, G. Styloglossus, H. Stylopharyngeus, I. Submandibular lymph nodes, J. Facial vein, K. Facial artery, L. Submental artery, M. Mylohyoid nerve and vessels, N. Superficial part of submandibular gland

**Practice Figure 4.3**

A. XII, B. XI, C. X, D. IX, E. Posterior auricular artery, F. Occipital artery, G. Internal carotid artery, H. Ascending pharyngeal artery, I. Outline of carotid triangle, J. Internal jugular vein, K. Styloid process, L. External carotid artery, M. Styloglossus, N. Stylohyoid ligament, O. Stylopharyngeus, P. Pharyngeal branch of vagus, Q. Facial artery, R. Lingual artery, T. Internal, U. External, V. Superior thyroid artery, W. Common carotid artery, X. Ansa cervicalis

**Practice Figure 4.4**

A. Meningeal branch C1, B. Inferior root (descendens cervicalis), C. To inferior belly of omohyoid, D. Ansa cervicalis, E. Hypoglossal nerve, F. Nerve to geniohyoid [C1], G. Nerve to thyrohyoid [C1], H. Superior root (descendens hypoglossi), I. To superior belly of omohyoid, J. To sternohyoid, K. To sternothyroid

### Key to MCQs

1. c  2. b  3. d  4. c  5. a  6. b  7. d
8. c  9. b  10. d  11. b  12. d

## Chapter 5

### Key to Clinicoanatomical Problem

#### *Clinical Case 1*

1. Acute parotitis is inflammation of the parotid gland due to infection or obstruction of its duct.
2. Increased pain during meals occurs because chewing stimulates saliva production from the parotid gland. In acute parotitis, increased saliva production during meals can exacerbate gland swelling and pain.
3. Because of inflammation causes the gland to swell, putting pressure on surrounding tissues and stretching the unyielding parotid fascia.
4. Mumps

### Key to Practice Figures

**Practice Figure 5.1**

A. IX, B. XII, C. XI, D. Internal carotid artery, E. Internal jugular vein, F. Posterior belly of digastric, G. Mastoid process, H. Sternocleidomastoid, I. External carotid artery, J. Retromandibular vein, K. Pharynx, L. Styloid apparatus, M. Medial pterygoid, N. Ramus of mandible, O. Masseter, P. Emerging branches of facial nerve, Q. Preauricular nodes, R. Superficial lamina of parotid fascia, S. Platysma, T. Superficial fascia with great auricular nerve, U. Skin

**Practice Figure 5.2**

A. Temporofacial trunk, B. Facial nerve trunk, C. Cervicofacial trunk, D. Superficial temporal vein, E. Retromandibular vein, F. Posterior division, G. Posterior auricular vein, H. External jugular vein, I. Posterior auricular artery, J. Temporal branch, K. Zygomatic branch, L. Upper buccal, M. Lower buccal, N. Marginal mandibular branch, O. Cervical branch, P. Transverse facial vein, Q. Maxillary vein, R. Anterior division, S. Facial vein, T. Common facial vein, U. Superficial temporal artery, V. Transverse facial artery, W. Maxillary artery, X. External carotid artery

### Key to MCQs

1. c  2. c  3. a  4. c  5. b  6. d  7. d
8. b  9. c  10. a  11. b  12. c

## Chapter 6

### Key to Clinicoanatomical Problems

#### Clinical Case 1

1. Anterior
2. The mandible is depressed posteriorly and inferiorly by exerting pressure on last molar teeth with thumbs and simultaneously the assistant elevates the chin.

#### Clinical Case 2

1. Because the tongue, lower jaw, and TMJ are supplied by mandibular division trigeminal nerve.

### Key to Practice Figures

#### Practice Figure 6.1

A. Deep temporal nerves, B. Deep temporal arteries, C. Masseteric nerve, D. Masseteric artery, E. Maxillary artery, F. Middle meningeal artery, G. Accessory meningeal artery, H. Pterygomaxillary fissure, I. Maxillary artery, J. Buccal artery, K. Buccal nerve, L. Lingual nerve, M. Inferior alveolar artery, N. Inferior alveolar nerve, 1. Deep auricular, 2. Anterior tympanic artery

#### Practice Figure 6.2

A. Accessory middle meningeal artery, B. Middle meningeal artery, C. Deep auricular artery, D. Anterior tympanic artery, E. Superficial temporal artery, F. Maxillary artery, G. Inferior alveolar artery, H. External carotid artery, I. Artery of pterygoid canal, J. Pharyngeal artery, K. Sphenopalatine artery, L. Greater palatine artery, M. Infraorbital artery, N. Posterior superior alveolar artery, O. Buccal artery, P. Pterygoid artery, Q. Masseteric artery, R. Incisive artery, S. Mental artery, T. Mylohyoid artery

#### Practice Figure 6.3

A. Articular fossa, B. Tympanic plate, C. Articular eminence, D. Upper compartment, E. Intra-articular disc, F. Lower compartment, G. Head of mandible

#### Practice Figure 6.4

A. Fibrous capsule, B. Styloid process, C. Articular tubercle, D. Lateral (temporomandibular) ligament, E. Sphenomandibular ligament, F. Lingula, G. Stylomandibular ligament

#### Practice Figure 6.5

A. Mandibular nerve (trunk, V3), B. Nervous spinosus, C. Middle meningeal artery, D. Auriculotemporal nerve, E. Chorda tympani nerve, F. Lingual nerve, G. Inferior alveolar nerve, H. Mylohyoid nerve, I. Nerve to medial pterygoid, J. Tensor tympani, K. Tensor veli palatini, L. Medial pterygoid, M. Otic ganglion, N. Deep temporal nerves, O. Masseteric nerve, P. Buccal nerve, Q. Nerve to lateral pterygoid, R. Submandibular ganglion, S. Incisive branch, T. Mental nerve, U. Nerve to mylohyoid muscle, V. Nerve to anterior belly of digastric muscle

### Key to MCQs

1. a  2. a  3. d  4. c  5. b  6. c  7. b
8. c  9. b  10. b  11. a

## Chapter 7

### Key to Clinicoanatomical Problem

#### Clinical Case 1

1. Pain increased during meals because chewing stimulates saliva production and stone obstructs the excretion of saliva. It increases the pressure that exacerbate the pain.
2. It allows the examiner to feel the gland between two hands: one hand inside the mouth and the other hand outside under the jaw.
3. Sialography is a radiographic technique used to visualise the salivary glands and their ducts by injecting a contrast dye into the duct.

### Key to Practice Figures

#### Practice Figure 7.1

A. Styloglossus, B. Glossopharyngeal nerve, C. Stylohyoid ligament, D. Middle constrictor of pharynx, E. Lingual artery, F. Hyoglossus, G. Genioglossus, H. Lingual nerves, I. Submandibular ganglion, J. Submandibular duct, K. Deep part of submandibular gland, L. Hypoglossal nerves and associated veins

#### Practice Figure 7.2

A. Anterior belly of digastric, B. Mylohyoid muscle, C. Superficial part, D. Deep part, E. Sublingual gland, F. Tongue, G. Hyoglossus

#### Practice Figure 7.3

A. Lingual nerve, B. Submandibular ganglion, C. Sublingual gland, D. Genioglossus, E. Submandibular duct, F. Hypoglossal nerve, G. Hyoglossus muscle, H. Deep part of submandibular gland

### Key to MCQs

1. c  2. a  3. c  4. a  5. a  6. b  7. d
8. c  9. b  10. c

## Chapter 8

### Key to Clinicoanatomical Problem

#### Clinical Case 1

1. A goitre is an abnormal enlargement of the thyroid gland. It may be due to iodine deficiency, autoimmune diseases, multinodular thyroid disease, and thyroid cancer.
2. Because the thyroid gland is attached to the trachea and larynx through the enclosing pretracheal fascia and ligament of Berry.
3. Due to compression of the recurrent laryngeal nerve, which supplies the vocal cords.

### Key to Practice Figures

#### Practice Figure 8.1

A. Hyoid bone, B. Thyroid cartilage, C. Levator glandulae thyroideae, D. Cricoid cartilage, E. Pyramidal lobe, F. First tracheal ring, G. Lateral lobe of thyroid gland, H. Isthmus of thyroid gland, I. Fifth tracheal ring

#### Practice Figure 8.2

A. Investing layer of deep cervical fascia, B. Pretracheal fascia, C. Carotid sheath, D. Prevertebral fascia, E. Trachea, F. Oesophagus, G. Sternohyoid, H. Sternothyroid, I. Omohyoid superior belly, J. Thyroid gland, K. Sternocleidomastoid, L. Recurrent laryngeal nerve, M. CCA, N. IJV, O. Vagus nerve, P. Sympathetic trunk, Q. Parathyroid gland

#### Practice Figure 8.3

A. Vagus nerve, B. External carotid artery, C. External laryngeal nerve, D. Superior thyroid artery, E. Anterior branch, F. Posterior branch, G. Inferior thyroid artery, H. Thyrocervical trunk, I. Subclavian artery, J. Recurrent laryngeal nerve, K. Arch of aorta, L. Superior laryngeal nerve, M. Thyroidea ima artery

#### Practice Figure 8.4

A. Styloid process, B. Styloglossus, C. Stylomandibular ligament, D. Stylohyoid ligament, E. Stylohyoid muscle, F. Stylopharyngeus, G. Tongue, H. Hyoid bone, I. Thyroid cartilage

### Key to MCQs

1. c  2. b  3. b  4. b  5. a  6. d  7. b
8. c  9. b  10. a  11. c  12. c

## Chapter 9

### Key to Clinicoanatomical Problems

#### Clinical Case 1

1. The fractured odontoid process damages the part of the brainstem that has cardiac and respiratory centres. It leads to death.
2. The headrest in a car prevents neck injuries during rear-end collisions. It prevents odontoid process fracture and death.
3. Apical ligament, alar ligaments, cruciate ligament.

*Clinical Case 2*

1. Due to the carcinoma of the oesophagus that caused obstruction of the oesophageal lumen.
2. Jugulodigastric, jugulo-omohyoid, supraclavicular, retropharyngeal nodes.
3. The carcinoma of the oesophagus causing compression of the recurrent laryngeal nerve which innervates the vocal cords, leading to hoarseness.

### Key to Practice Figures

**Practice Figure 9.1**

A. Basilar artery, B. Fourth part of vertebral artery, C. Foramen magnum, D. Third part of vertebral artery, E. Transverse process of atlas, F. Second part of vertebral artery, G. Transverse process of C6, H. First part of vertebral artery, I. 1st part of subclavian artery

**Practice Figure 9.2**

A. Lesser occipital (C2), B. Greater auricular (C2, C3), C. Spinal accessory nerve, D. Fibres of C2, C3, C4, E. Suprascapular nerve (C3–C4), F. Dorsal scapular nerve (nerve to levator scapulae, C3–C5), G. To rectus capitis anterior (C1), H. Meningeal branch (C1), I. Hypoglossal nerve, J. Nerve to geniohyoid (C1), K. Nerve to thyrohyoid (C1), L. To rectus capitis lateralis (C2, C3), M. Superior root (descendens hypoglossi), N. Inferior root (descendens cervicalis), O. To superior belly of omohyoid, P. To sternohyoid, Q. To sternothyroid, R. To inferior belly of omohyoid, S. Phrenic nerve (C3–C5)

### Key to MCQs

| | | | | | | |
|---|---|---|---|---|---|---|
| 1. c | 2. a | 3. c | 4. d | 5. a | 6. b | 7. b |
| 8. a | 9. c | 10. d | 11. a | | | |

## Chapter 10

### Key to Clinicoanatomical Problem

*Clinical Case 1*

1. A sore throat, or pharyngitis, is inflammation of the pharynx, commonly caused by viral or bacterial infections.
2. The sore throat likely led to meningitis through the spread of infection via the bloodstream or through the middle ear cavity.
3. Neck stiffness in meningitis is due to inflammation of the meninges, causing irritation and spasm of the neck muscles, leading to characteristic nuchal rigidity. This occurs due to irritation of the spinal accessory nerve and C1 to C3 nerves.
4. CSF collection in the neck is performed via a cisternal puncture by passing a needle through the posterior side of the neck between the occipital bone and C1 vertebra.

### Key to Practice Figure

**Practice Figure 10.1**

A. Posterior atlanto-occipital membrane, B. Rectus capitis posterior minor, C. Rectus capitis posterior major, D. Semispinalis capitis, E. Obliquus capitis superior, F. Vertebral artery (3rd part), G. Suboccipital nerve (dorsal ramus of C1), H. Obliquus capitis inferior, I. Greater occipital nerve (medial branch of dorsal ramus of C2), J. Vertebral artery (2nd part)

### Key to MCQs

| | | | | | | |
|---|---|---|---|---|---|---|
| 1. a | 2. c | 3. c | 4. d | 5. b | 6. d | 7. a |
| 8. a | 9. d | 10. b | | | | |

## Chapter 11

### Key to Clinicoanatomical Problem

*Clinical Case 1*

1. The veins from prostate drain into prostatic venous plexus which communicates with the pelvic veins. These veins communicates with the vertebral venous plexus of Batson which continues up the whole height of the vertebral canal and drains into segmental veins in abdominal cavity, thoracic cavity, in the neck and in basilar venous plexus. This plexus is valveless. The cancer cells 'climb' up through this plexus from the prostatic cancer to the cervical vertebrae and the brain.

### Key to Practice Figures

**Practice Figure 11.1**

A. Ligamentum denticulatum, B. Dura mater, C. Subdural space, D. Arachnoid mater, E. Nerve roots, F. Subarachnoid space, G. Pia mater, H. Space for spinal cord

**Practice Figure 11.2**

A. Dura mater, B. Arachnoid mater, C. Subarachnoid septum, D. Pia mater, E. Subarachnoid space, F. Dorsal nerve root, G. Spinal ganglion, I. Nerve trunk, H. Dorsal ramus, J. Ventral nerve root, K. Ligamentum denticulatum, L. Subdural space, M. Linea splendens, N. Internal vertebral venous plexus

### Key to MCQs

| | | | | | | |
|---|---|---|---|---|---|---|
| 1. c | 2. d | 3. c | 4. d | 5. a | 6. b | 7. c |
| 8. c | 9. c | 10. b | 11. b | | | |

## Chapter 12

### Key to Clinicoanatomical Problems

*Clinical Case 1*

1. The carotid-cavernous fistula (CCF) is an abnormal connection between the carotid artery and the cavernous sinus.
2. Pulsating exophthalmos occurs because of the abnormal connection between the carotid artery and the cavernous sinus. The causes increased pressure in the veins of orbit, protrusion of the eyeball (exophthalmos) and the pulsation that synchronizes with the arterial pulse.

*Clinical Case 2*

1. Because the pituitary tumour compresses the optic chiasma, where the nasal fibres of the optic nerves from both eyes cross.
2. Tubular vision occurred as the peripheral vision is lost due to the compression of the optic chiasma by the pituitary tumour.

### Key to Practice Figures

**Practice Figure 12.1**

A. Optic nerve, B. Anterior clinoid process, C. Internal carotid artery, D. Trigeminal ganglion in trigeminal cave, E. Great cerebral vein, F. Straight sinus, G. Infundibulum, H. Free margin of tentorium cerebelli, I. Oculomotor nerve, J. Trochlear nerve, K. Superior petrosal sinus, L. Tentorium cerebelli, M. Transverse sinus

**Practice Figure 12.2**

A. Optic tract, B. Hypophysis cerebri, C. Arachnoid mater, D. Meningeal dura mater, E. Endothelium, F. Endosteal layer of dura mater, G. Sphenoidal air sinus, H. Internal carotid artery, I. Abducent nerve, J. Internal carotid artery, K. Oculomotor nerve, L. Trochlear nerve, M. Ophthalmic nerve, N. Mandibular nerve

**Practice Figure 12.3**

A. Posterior intercavernous sinus, B. Anterior intercavernous sinus, C. Sphenoparietal sinus, D. Fontal (anterior) trunk of middle meningeal vein, E. Inferior cerebral veins, F. Basilar plexus of veins, G. Internal jugular vein, H. Connection with internal venous plexus, I. Occipital sinus, J. Inferior cerebral veins, K. Cavernous sinus, L. Superficial middle cerebral vein, M. Superior petrosal sinus, N. Inferior petrosal sinus, O. Sigmoid sinus, P. Transverse sinus, Q. Confluence of sinuses

### Key to MCQs

| | | | | | | |
|---|---|---|---|---|---|---|
| 1. c | 2. b | 3. a | 4. a | 5. b | 6. b | 7. d |
| 8. c | 9. b | 10. d | 11. b | 12. b | | |

## Chapter 13

### Key to Clinicoanatomical Problems

#### *Clinical Case 1*

1. Due to the unopposed action of the lateral rectus and superior oblique muscles.
2. Because the oculomotor nerve palsy impaired the medial rectus (adductor of eyeball) and superior rectus muscles (elevates the eye and turns it slightly inward).
3. The patient had ptosis and a dilated pupil due to the involvement of the levator palpebrae superioris muscle and the pupillary sphincter muscle, both of which are innervated by the parasympathetic fibres of oculomotor nerve.

#### *Clinical Case 2*

1. Hypertension causes atheromatous changes in the central artery of the retina which is an 'end artery' with no anastomoses.
2. Central artery of retina, labyrinthine artery for the inner ear, central branches of cerebral arteries, segmental branches of the kidney and spleen.

### Key to Practice Figures

**Practice Figure 13.1**

A. Lesser wing of sphenoid, B. Superior rectus, C. Lacrimal nerve, D. Frontal nerve, E. Trochlear nerve, F. Superior ophthalmic vein, G. Upper division of oculomotor nerve, H. Nasociliary nerve, I. Lower division of oculomotor nerve, J. Abducent nerve, K. Inferior ophthalmic vein, L. Levator palpebrae superioris, M. Common tendinous ring, N. Superior oblique, O. Body of sphenoid, P. Medial rectus, Q. Optic nerve with central artery of retina, R. Ophthalmic artery, S. Inferior rectus, T. Lateral rectus

**Practice Figure 13.2**

A. Levator palpebrae superioris, B. Superior rectus, C. Upper division of oculomotor nerve, D. Lateral rectus, E. Abducent nerve, F. Ciliary ganglion, G. Trochlear nerve, H. Superior oblique, I. Medial rectus, J. Lower division of oculomotor nerve, K. Inferior rectus, L. Inferior oblique, M. Optic canal, N. Nasociliary nerve

**Practice Figure 13.3**

1. Inferior oblique, 2. Superior rectus, 3. Lateral rectus, 4. Medial rectus, 5. Superior oblique, 6. Inferior rectus

### Key to MCQs

1. b  2. c  3. c  4. c  5. a  6. b  7. a
8. d  9. c  10. b

## Chapter 14

### Key to Clinicoanatomical Problems

#### *Clinical Case 1*

1. Palatine tonsils, pharyngeal tonsil (adenoids), lingual tonsils, tubal tonsils
2. The earache in tonsillitis is due to referred pain through the common nerve supply – glossopharyngeal nerve.
3. Tonsillectomy.
4. Jugulodigastric lymph node, also known as the tonsillar node.

#### *Clinical Case 2*

1. A small, pear-shaped recess located in the laryngopharynx on either side of the laryngeal opening.
2. Internal laryngeal branch of the superior laryngeal nerve, a branch of the vagus nerve.
3. Smuggler's fossa.

### Key to Practice Figures

**Practice Figure 14.1**

A. Enamel, B. Dentine, C. Pulp cavity, D. Gum, E. Cement, F. Odontoblasts, G. Periodontal membrane, H. Alveolar bone, I. Apical foramen

**Practice Figure 14.2**

A. Pterygoid hamulus, B. Palatine aponeurosis, C. Musculus uvulae, D. Levator veli palatini, E. Tensor veli palatini, F. Palatopharyngeus, G. Palatoglossus

**Practice Figure 14.3**

A. Auditory tube, B. Styloid process, C. Stylopharyngeus, D. Glossopharyngeal nerve, E. Branch to stylopharyngeus, F. Middle constrictor, G. Internal laryngeal nerve, H. Superior laryngeal vessels, I. Inferior constrictor, J. Inferior laryngeal vessels, K. Recurrent laryngeal nerve, L. Levator palati, M. Ascending palatine artery, N. Superior constrictor

**Practice Figure 14.4**

A. Paratonsillar vein, B. Pharyngobasilar fascia, C. Superior constrictor, D. Buccopharyngeal fascia, E. Styloglossus, F. Glossopharyngeal nerve, G. Peritonsillar space, H. Palatopharyngeus muscle, I. Palatopharyngeal arch, J. Intratonsillar cleft, K. Tonsillar crypts, L. Palatine tonsil, M. Palatoglossal arch, N. Palatoglossus muscle

### Key to MCQs

1. a  2. d  3. b  4. b  5. c  6. d  7. b
8. b  9. d  10. b  11. b  12. b  13. c

## Chapter 15

### Key to Clinicoanatomical Problem

#### *Clinical Case 1*

1. Located in the anteroinferior part of the nasal septum, also known as Little's area.
2. Anterior ethmoidal artery, sphenopalatine artery, greater palatine artery, superior labial artery, and septal branch of the posterior ethmoidal artery (a branch of the ophthalmic artery)
3. Sphenopalatine artery.

### Key to Practice Figures

**Practice Figure 15.1**

A. Sphenopalatine artery, B. Posterior ethmoidal artery, C. Anterior ethmoidal artery, D. Little's area, E. Superior labial artery, F. Greater palatine artery

**Practice Figure 15.2**

A. Frontal sinus, B. Middle concha, C. Agger nasi, D. Atrium, E. Hiatus semilunaris, F. Vestibule, G. Opening of nasolacrimal duct, H. Inferior meatus, I. Inferior concha, J. Opening of frontal sinus in the infundibulum, K. Opening of anterior ethmoidal sinus, L. Sphenoethmoidal recess, M. Sphenoidal sinus, N. Superior concha, O. Opening of posterior ethmoidal sinus, P. Opening of middle ethmoidal sinus on ethmoidal bulla, Q. Opening of maxillary sinus

**Practice Figure 15.3**

A. Medial posterior superior nasal branches of pterygopalatine ganglion, B. Nasopalatine nerve from pterygopalatine ganglion, C. Olfactory nerves, D. Internal nasal branch of anterior ethmoidal nerve, E. Anterior superior alveolar nerve

### Key to MCQs

1. d  2. d  3. b  4. c  5. d  6. a  7. c
8. d  9. a  10. d  11. a

## Chapter 16

### Key to Clinicoanatomical Problem

#### *Clinical Case 1*

1. Because of obstructed airway by the inhaled foreign body.
2. It is a first aid procedure to dislodge foreign objects from the upper respiratory tract by applying abdominal thrusts.
3. Glottis (between the vocal cords).

### Key to Practice Figures

**Practice Figure 16.1**

A. Opening for superior laryngeal vessels and internal laryngeal nerve, B. Epiglottis, C. Hyoid bone, D. Thyrohyoid membrane, E. Lateral thyrohyoid ligament, F. Cartilago triticea, G. Median thyroid ligament, H. Superior cornu of thyroid, I. Thyroid cartilage, J. Cricothyroid membrane, K. Inferior cornu of thyroid, L. Cricothyroid ligament, M. Arch of cricoid cartilage, N. Cricotracheal membrane

**Practice Figure 16.2**

A. Quadrangular (quadrate) membrane, B. Cuneiform cartilage, C. Corniculate cartilage, D. Arytenoid cartilage, E. Epiglottis, F. Hyoepiglottic ligament, G. Pre-epiglottic space, H. Hyoid bone, I. Subhyoid bursa, J. Thyrohyoid membrane, K. Thyroepiglottic ligament, L. Vestibular ligament, M. Vocal ligament, N. Cricothyroid membrane, O. Cricovocal membrane, P. Cricoid cartilage

### Key to MCQs

1. c 2. a 3. b 4. c 5. a 6. c 7. c
8. b 9. b 10. c 11. d 12. b

## Chapter 17

### Key to Clinicoanatomical Problem

#### *Clinical Case 1*

1. Facial nerve.
2. a. Chorda tympani nerve carries taste sensation from the anterior two-thirds of the tongue, and its injury can lead to altered taste perception.
   b. Damage to chorda tympani nerve result into loss of parasympathetic supply to submandibular and sublingual glands and dryness of mouth.

### Key to Practice Figures

**Practice Figure 17.1**

A. Median fibrous septum, B. Greater cornu of hyoid bone, C. Superior longitudinal muscle, D. Vertical, E. Transverse, F. Inferior longitudinal muscle, G. Styloglossus, H. Genioglossus, I. Hyoglossus muscles

**Practice Figure 17.2**

A. Hypoglossal nerve all muscles except palatoglossus, B. Posteriormost part of tongue, fourth arch, general and special sensory: Superior laryngeal branch of vagus nerve, C. Posterior 1/3rd of tongue and circumvallate papillae, third arch, general and special sensory: Glossopharyngeal nerve, D. Anterior 2/3rds of tongue, first arch, special sensory: Chorda tympani branch of facial nerve, general sensory: Lingual branch of mandibular nerve

**Practice Figure 17.3**

A. Epiglottis, B. Median glossoepiglottic fold, C. Palato-pharyngeal fold, D. Palatine tonsil, E. Palato-glossal fold, F. Foliate papillae, G. Filiform papillae, H. Vallecula of epiglottis, I. Lateral glossoepiglottic fold, J. Lymphoid nodules on pharyngeal part of the dorsum, K. Foramen caecum, L. Sulcus terminalis, M. Vallate papillae, N. Fungiform papillae

### Key to MCQs

1. d 2. b 3. a 4. b 5. a 6. b 7. b
8. c 9. b 10. b 11. b 12. b

## Chapter 18

### Key to Clinicoanatomical Problem

#### *Clinical Case 1*

1. Otitis media is an inflammation or infection of the middle ear.
2. Through the Eustachian tube.
3. Normal findings during an otoscopy include: Semi-transparent oval tympanic membrane, umbo, handle of malleus, long process of incus, and cone of light.

### Key to Practice Figures

**Practice Figure 18.1**

A. Pars flaccida (Shrapnell's membrane), B. Posterior malleolar fold, C. Long process of incus (lower half), D. Pars tensa, E. Site of myringotomy, F. Lateral process of malleus, G. Anterior malleolar fold, H. Handle of malleus, I. Umbo, J. Cone of light

**Practice Figure 18.2**

A. Prominence of lateral semicircular canal, B. Prominence of facial canal (oblique part), C. Aditus ad antrum, D. Malleus, E. Medial aspect of tympanic membrane, F. Pyramid with stapedius, G. Chorda tympani nerve, H. Tympanic branch of glossopharyngeal nerve, I. Facial canal, J. Bulb of internal jugular vein, K. Oval window, L. Tegmen tympani, M. Pulley, N. Processus cochleariformis, O. Canal for tensor tympani, P. Tubal opening, Q. Incus

**Practice Figure 18.3**

A. Mastoid antrum, B. Aditus ad antrum, C. Tegmen tympani, D. Auditory tube, E. Mastoid air cells, F. Mastoid process, G. Middle ear

### Key to MCQs

1. a 2. c 3. d 4. a 5. d 6. d 7. c
8. b 9. b 10. c 11. a 12. d

## Chapter 19

### Key to Clinicoanatomical Problem

#### *Clinical Case 1*

1. The retinal detachment is actually an inter retinal detachment. The outer pigmented layer stays with choroid, while the inner nine layers get detached and cause the problem.
2. Central retinal artery which is the branch of the ophthalmic artery.
3. Optic disc is a white spot about 3 mm medial to the macula. The nerve fibres from retina converge and pass through the optic disc of the eyeball to form the optic nerve. The blood vessels of retina also pass through the optic disc.

### Key to Practice Figures

**Practice Figure 19.1**

A. Pupil, B. Cornea, C. Iris, D. Conjunctiva, E. Ciliary zonule, F. Hyaloid canal, G. Optic stalk, H. Optic nerve, I. Anterior chamber, J. Posterior chamber, K. Ciliary body, L. Lens, M. Visual axis, N. Sclera, O. Choroid, P. Retina, Q. Fovea centralis, R. Vitreous body

**Practice Figure 19.2**

A. Corneal epithelium, B. Bowman's layer, C. Stroma, D. Descemet's membrane, E. Corneal endothelium

### Key to MCQs

1. c 2. c 3. c 4. b 5. b 6. c 7. b
8. c 9. c 10. d 11. b 12. d

## Chapter 20

### Key to Practice Figures

**Practice Figure 20.1**

A. External acostic meatus, B. C1, C. Frontal air sinus, D. Maxillary sinus

**Practice Figure 20.2**

A. Frontal sinus, B. Ethmoidal air sinus, C. Maxillary sinus, D. Nasal septum, E. Alveolar process of maxilla

### Key to MCQs

1. c 2. d 3. b 4. b 5. c 6. a 7. b
8. a 9. b 10. a 11. c

# BRAIN–NEUROANATOMY

## Chapter 1

### Key to Clinicoanatomical Problem

#### *Clinical Case 1*

1. From the site of the wound, the rabies virus reaches the brain from the lower limb through axonal transport within the peripheral nerves.
2. Using anti-rabies vaccine.

## Key to Practice Figure

### Practice Figure 1.1

A. Multipolar, B. Nissl granules, C. Axon hillock, D. Node of Ranvier, E. Dendrites, F. Soma (perikaryon), G. Nucleus, H. Myelin sheath, I. Axon, J. Axolemma, K. Schwann cell (neurolemmocytes), L. Axon terminal

## Key to MCQs

1. d 2. d 3. d 4. c 5. d 6. d 7. d
8. d 9. a 10. b 11. d 12. b 13. a

# Chapter 2

## Key to Clinicoanatomical Problems

### *Clinical Case 1*

1. a. In neurotmesis – both axon and myelin sheath damaged.
   b. In axonotmesis – only axon is damaged, myelin sheath is intact.
   c. In neuropraxia – both axon and myelin sheath are preserved.

### *Clinical Case 2*

1. Peripheral neuropathy is a disease or injury that affects the functions of the peripheral nerve.
   It may have acute (rapid) onset or chronic (slower onset) progressive course.
2. Peripheral neuropathy disrupts the normal signalling pathways, leading to a loss of sensation in the affected areas.

## Key to Practice Figure

### Practice Figure 2.1

A. Nissl granules, B. Schwann cell, C. Axon, D. Site of injury, E. Chromatolysis, F. Phagocytes removing debris, G. Eccentric nucleus, H. Axon fragments, I. Retrograde degeneration, J. Proliferating Schwann cells, K. Axonal sprouts

## Key to MCQs

1. c 2. d 3. c 4. a 5. d 6. a 7. a
8. a 9. a 10. a

# Chapter 3

## Key to Clinicoanatomical Problem

### *Clinical Case 1*

a. Organophosphorus poisoning causes overstimulation of the parasympathetic nervous system, resulting in constriction of the pupils.
b. The accumulation of acetylcholine at muscarinic receptors also stimulates the salivary glands excessively, leading to increased salivation.
c. Organophosphorus compounds bind to and inhibit the action of acetylcholinesterase. As a result, acetylcholine accumulates in the synaptic cleft causing continuous stimulation of muscle fibres. This eventually causes fatigue and paralysis of the respiratory muscles, leading to respiratory failure.

## Key to Practice Figure

### Practice Figure 3.1

A. Neurotendinous spindles, B. Neuromuscular spindles, C. Motor end plates, D. Afferent neuron, E. Alpha (α) motor neuron

## Key to MCQs

1. c 2. d 3. c 4. a 5. a 6. b 7. d
8. a 9. a 10. d

# Chapter 4

## Key to Clinicoanatomical Problem

### *Clinical Case 1*

1. Hydrocephalus is an accumulation of cerebrospinal fluid (CSF) within the ventricles of the brain.
2. The enlargement of ventricles in hydrocephalus increases intracranial pressure, causing the infant's skull to expand since the sutures and fontanelles are not yet fused. This leads to an abnormally large head and bulging fontanelles.
3. It is the largest cistern lying in the angle between medulla oblongata, cerebellum and occipital bone.

## Key to Practice Figures

### Practice Figure 4.1

A. Falx cerebri, B. Falx cerebelli, C. Diaphragma sellae, D. Tentorium cerebelli

### Practice Figure 4.2

A. Subarachnoid space, B. Foramen of Monro, C. Interpeduncular cistern, D. Cerebral aqueduct of sylvius, E. Cisterna pontis, F. Arachnoid granulation, G. Choroid plexus, H. Lateral ventricle (dotted outline), I. Superior sagittal sinus, J. 3rd ventricle, K. Great cerebral vein of Galen, L. Cistern of great cerebral vein (cisterna ambiens), M. Foramen of Luschka, N. 4th ventricle, O. Foramen of Magendie, P. Cerebellomedullary cistern (cisterna magna), Q. Central canal, R. Terminal ventricle, S. Lumbar cistern, T. Filum terminale

## Key to MCQs

1. b 2. c 3. a 4. c 5. d 6. a 7. b
8. a 9. c 10. c 11. a 12. b

# Chapter 5

## Key to Clinicoanatomical Problems

### *Clinical Case 1*

1. Upper motor neuron paralysis.
2. Babinski's sign is a plantar reflex characterised by the dorsiflexion of the big toe and fanning of the other toes in response to the stimulation of the sole of the foot. Abnormal Babinski's sign indicates upper motor neuron damage.
3. In the upper motor neurons are paralysis, their inhibitory influence is reduced, leading to unopposed activity of lower motor neurons and subsequent increased muscle tone.

### *Clinical Case 2*

1. Cauda equina syndrome
2. Due to the cauda equina nerve roots, which control bladder function.

## Key to Practice Figures

### Practice Figure 5.1

A. Anterior median fissure, B. Anterolateral sulcus, C. Medulla oblongata, D. Cervical enlargement (C4 to T2), E. Posterior intermediate sulcus, F. Posterolateral sulcus, G. Posterior median sulcus, H. Lumbar enlargement (L2 to S3), I. Conus medullaris, J. Filum terminale internum, K. Filum terminale externum

### Practice Figure 5.2

A. Dorsal grey commissure, B. Posterolateral sulcus, C. Posterior horn, D. Lateral horn, E. Anterior horn, F. Ventral grey commissure, G. Anterior median fissure, H. Posterior median sulcus, I. Posterior median septum, J. Posterior funiculus, K. Lateral funiculus, L. Central canal, M. Anterolateral sulcus, N. White commissure, O. Anterior funiculus

### Practice Figure 5.3

A. Postero-intermediate sulcus, B. Long and slender posterior horn, C. Broad and massive anterior horn, D. Slender posterior horn, E. Lateral horn, F. Slender anterior horn, G. Bulbous and short posterior horn, H. Bulbous and short anterior horn, I. Thick posterior horn, J. Broad anterior horn

### Practice Figure 5.4

A. Midbrain, B. Pons, C. Medulla oblongata, D. Anterior corticospinal tract (uncrossed), E. Spinal cord, F. Motor cortex (precentral gyrus, Area 4), G. Corona radiata, H. Internal capsule, I. Upper motor neuron, J. Crus cerebri, K. Basilar part, L. Pyramid, M. Pyramidal decussation (75–90% fibres cross), N. Lateral corticospinal tract (crossed), O. Lower motor neuron

**Practice Figure 5.5**

A. Posteromarginal nucleus, B. Substantia gelatinosa, C. Nucleus proprius, D. Nucleus dorsalis (Clarke's column), E. Visceral afferent nucleus, F. Intermediolateral nucleus, G. Intermediomedial nucleus, H. Lateral group, I. Central group, J. Medial group

**Practice Figure 5.6**

A. Thalamus, B. Passes through brainstem, C. Lateral spinothalamic tract, D. Spinal cord, E. Primary sensory cortex, F. 3rd order neuron, G. Ventral posterolateral nucleus, H. 1st order neuron, I. Central process, J. Peripheral process, K. Sensory inputs, L. Dorsal root ganglion, M. 2nd order neuron

**Practice Figure 5.7**

A. Thalamus, B. Passes through brainstem, C. Spinal cord, D. Anterior spinothalamic tract, E. Primary sensory cortex, F. 3rd order neuron, G. Ventral posterolateral nucleus, H. 1st order neuron, I. Central process, J. Peripheral process, K. Sensory inputs, L. Dorsal root ganglion, M. 2nd order neuron

**Practice Figure 5.8**

A. Thalamus, B. Medial lemniscus, C. Nucleus gracilis, D. Fasciculus gracilis, E. Fasciculus cuneatus, F. Spinal cord, G. Primary sensory cortex, H. 3rd order neuron, I. Ventral posterolateral nucleus, J. 2nd order neuron, K. Nucleus cuneatus, L. 1st order neuron, M. Central process, N. Peripheral process, O. Sensory inputs, P. Dorsal root ganglion

### Key to MCQs

| | | | | | | |
|---|---|---|---|---|---|---|
| 1. d | 2. b | 3. b | 4. a | 5. a | 6. a | 7. a |
| 8. c | 9. d | 10. d | 11. a | 12. c | | |

## Chapter 6

### Key to Clinicoanatomical Problems

#### Clinical Case 1

1. Because of the paralysis of the right abducens nerve which innervates the lateral rectus muscle, and the unopposed action of the medial rectus muscle pulls the eye medially.
2. Due to its long intracranial course and its crossing over the petrous part of temporal bone. Increased intracranial pressure cause downward displacement of the brainstem and stretching of the abducens nerve which lead to its paralysis.

#### Clinical Case 2

1. Right oculomotor nerve
2. Right midbrain at the level of superior colliculus
3. Due to the involvement of the parasympathetic fibres of the Edinger-Westphal nucleus which innervate the sphincter pupillae muscle.

#### Clinical Case 3

1. Because the motor nucleus of facial nerve receives bilateral cortical input for the muscles of the upper face.
2. Because the corticonuclear fibres from the left cerebral cortex decussate and control the right facial nerve nucleus.

### Key to Practice Figures

**Practice Figure 6.1**

A. Orbit, B. Superior oblique (SO4), C. Medial rectus, D. Inferior rectus, E. Inferior oblique, F. Lower division, G. Oculomotor nerve, H. Midbrain, I. Levator palpebrae superioris, J. Superior rectus, K. Lateral rectus (LR6), L. Ciliary ganglion, M. Upper division, N. Superior orbital fissure, O. Cavernous sinus, P. Posterior cerebral artery, Q. Superior cerebellar artery, R. Oculomotor nucleus, S. Periaqueductal grey matter

**Practice Figure 6.2**

A. Nervus spinosus, B. Auriculotemporal nerve, C. Middle meningeal artery, D. Chorda tympani nerve, E. Lingual nerve, F. Inferior alveolar nerve, G. Mylohyoid nerve, H. Mandibular nerve (trunk, V3), I. Nerve to medial pterygoid, J. Tensor tympani, K. Tensor veli palatini, L. Medial pterygoid, M. Otic ganglion, N. Deep temporal nerves, O. Masseteric nerve, P. Buccal nerve, Q. Nerve to lateral pterygoid, R. Submandibular ganglion, S. Incisive branch, T. Mental nerve, U. Nerve to mylohyoid muscle, V. Nerve to anterior belly of digastric muscle

**Practice Figure 6.3**

A. Orbit, B. Superior oblique (SO4), C. Medial rectus, D. Inferior rectus, E. Inferior oblique, F. Pons, G. Levator palpebrae superioris, H. Superior rectus, I. Lateral rectus (LR6), J. Abducent nerve, K. Superior orbital fissure, L. Cavernous sinus, M. Anterior inferior cerebellar artery, N. Motor nucleus of facial nerve, O. Abducent nucleus, P. Facial colliculus

**Practice Figure 6.4**

A. Abducent nucleus, B. Superior salivatory and lacrimatory nuclei, C. Nucleus tractus solitarius, D. Spinal nucleus of trigeminal nerve, E. Motor nucleus of facial nerve, F. GSA: Ear, G. SVA: Taste, H. SVE: Muscles of 2nd pharyngeal arch, I. Pons, J. Facial nerve, K. GVE: Lacrimal, submandibular and sublingual salivary glands

**Practice Figure 6.5**

A. SVED. B. Nucleus ambiguus, C. Foramen magnum, D. Spinal nucleus of accessory nerve, E. GSE, F. Accessory nerve, G. Sternocleidomastoid, H. Trapezius, I. Roots of accessory nerve, J. Cranial root, K. Spinal root, L. Vagus nerve, M. Muscles of palate, N. Muscles of pharynx, O. Muscles of larynx

### Key to MCQs

| | | | | | | |
|---|---|---|---|---|---|---|
| 1. b | 2. c | 3. b | 4. a | 5. b | 6. c | 7. c |
| 8. d | 9. a | 10. b | 11. d | 12. c | 13. b | 14. b |

## Chapter 7

### Key to Clinicoanatomical Problems

#### Clinical Case 1

1. A midbrain infarct affecting the cerebral peduncle and oculomotor nerve fibres.
2. Posterior cerebral artery.
3. Right corticospinal fibres.

#### Clinical Case 2

a. Pontine haemorrhage disrupted the hypothalamic thermo-regulatory centres, leading to uncontrolled hyperpyrexia.
b. Loss of consciousness occurred due to the extensive damage to ascending reticular system which is located in the brainstem.
c. The pinpoint pupils resulted from dysfunction of the para-sympathetic fibres carried by the oculomotor nerve.

### Key to Practice Figures

**Practice Figure 7.1**

A. Fasciculus gracilis, B. Fasciculus cuneatus, C. Reticular formation, D. Nucleus gracilis, E. Nucleus cuneatus, F. Spinal tract, G. Spinal nucleus, H. Lateral corticospinal tract, I. Dorsal, J. Ventral, K. Spino-cerebellar tracts, L. Lateral spinothalamic tract, M. Detached anterior horn, N. Pyramidal decussation, O. Pyramid

**Practice Figure 7.2**

A. Central grey matter, B. Nucleus tractus solitarius, C. Dorsal nucleus of vagus, D. Hypoglossal nucleus, E. Reticular formation, F. Medial longitudinal bundle, G. Inferior olivary nucleus, H. Nucleus gracilis, I. Nucleus cuneatus, J. Accessory cuneate nuleus, K. Spinal tract, L. Spinal nucleus, M. of trigeminal nerve, N. Dorsal, O. Ventral, P. Spino-cerebellar tracts, Q. Lateral spinothalamic tract, R. Internal arcuate fibres, S. Medial lemniscus, T. Pyramid

**Practice Figure 7.3**

A. Inferior medullary velum, B. Dorsal nucleus of vagus, C. Dorsal cochlear nucleus, D. Nucleus of tractus solitarius, E. Hypoglossal nucleus, F. Nucleus ambiguus, G. Ventral cochlear nucleus, H. Dorsal, I. Medial, J. Accessory olivary nuclei, K. Inferior olivary nucleus, L. Arcuate nucleus, M. Medial, N. Inferior, O. Vestibular nuclei, P. Inferior cerebellar peduncle,

Q. Spinal tract, R. Spinal nucleus, S. of trigeminal nerve, T. Lateral spinothalamic track, U. Vagus nerve, V. Medial lemniscus, W. Pyramidal tract, X. Hypoglossal nerve

### Practice Figure 7.4

A. Abducent nucleus, B. Vestibular nuclei, C. Dorsal, D. Ventral, E. Cochlear nuclei, F. Motor nucleus of facial nerve, G. Pontine nuclei, H. Internal genu of facial nerve, I. Inferior cerebellar peduncle, J. Middle cerebellar peduncle, K. Spinal tract, L. Spinal nucleus, M. of trigeminal nerve, N. Superior salivatory nucleus, O. Facial nerve, P. Spinal lemniscus, Q. Medial lemniscus, R. Trapezoid body, S. Transverse pontocerebellar fibres, T. Longitudinal bundles of corticonuclear and corticospinal fibres, U. Abducent nerve, V. Facial colliculus

### Practice Figure 7.5

A. Motor nucleus of trigeminal nerve, B. Main sensory nucleus of trigeminal nerve, C. Pontine nuclei, D. Superior medullary velum, E. Superior cerebellar peduncle, F. Middle cerebellar peduncle, G. Transverse pontocerebellar fibres, H. Longitudinal bundles of corticonuclear and corticospinal fibres, I. Trigeminal nerve, J. Lateral, K. Spinal, L. Trigeminal, M. Medial, N. Lemnisci (MTSL), O. 4th ventricle

### Practice Figure 7.6

A. Trochlear nerve, B. Nucleus of inferior colliculus, C. Mesencephalic nucleus of trigeminal nerve, D. Trochlear nerve nucleus, E. Midbrain reticular formation, F. Lateral, G. Spinal, H. Trigeminal, I. Medial, J. Lemnisci, K. Temporopontine, parietopontine and occipitopontine fibres (lateral 1/6th), L. Corticonuclear and corticospinal fibres of pyramidal tract (middle 2/3rd), M. Frontopontine fibres (medial 1/6th), N. Decussation of superior cerebellar peduncles

### Practice Figure 7.7

A. Nucleus of superior colliculus, B. Pretectal nucleus, C. Mesencephalic nucleus of trigeminal nerve, D. Oculomotor nucleus, E. Midbrain reticular formation, F. Red nucleus, G. Oculomotor nerve, H. Median longitudinal bundle, I. Spinal, J. Trigeminal, K. Medial, L. Lemnisci, M. Dorsal tegmental decussation (of Meynert), N. Ventral tegmental decussation (of Forel), O. Temporopontine, parietopontine and occipitopontine fibres (lateral 1/6th), P. Corticonuclear and corticospinal fibres of pyramidal tract (middle 2/3rd), Q. Frontopontine fibres (medial 1/6th)

## Key to MCQs

1. a 2. b 3. d 4. c 5. a 6. d 7. c
8. d 9. b 10. a 11. d 12. d 13. a 14. d
15. c 16. b 17. d 18. b 19. d 20. c

## Chapter 8

## Key to Clinicoanatomical Problems

### Clinical Case 1

1. Vermis syndrome
2. Truncal ataxia refers to difficulty maintaining balance while sitting or standing, often resulting in a swaying or staggering gait.
3. Dysmetria involves inaccurate estimation or control of movements, typically affecting the limbs.

### Clinical Case 2

1. Asynergy: Loss of smooth movements. The movements are intermittent and jerky.
2. Intention tremors are the tremors that come on initiation of voluntary movement and disappear during rest.
3. Dysarthria or scanning speech is the muscular incoordination that produces slurred, prolonged, explosive speech with pause in wrong place.

## Key to Practice Figure

### Practice Figure 8.1

A. Superior surface, B. Inferior surface, C. Fissura prima, D. Horizontal fissure, E. Posterolateral fissure, F. Nodule, G. Lingula, H. Anterior lobe, I. Posterior or middle lobe, J. Flocculonodular lobe, K. Flocculus

## Key to MCQs

1. a 2. b 3. b 4. c 5. d 6. b 7. a
8. d 9. c 10. a 11. a

## Chapter 9

## Key to Clinicoanatomical Problem

### Clinical Case 1

1. Hydrocephalus is an abnormal accumulation of cerebrospinal fluid (CSF) within the ventricles of the brain.
2. Lesions of the fourth ventricle can obstruct the foramen of Magendie and foramen of Luschka which are important sites of escape for CSF from the ventricle to the subarachnoid space.

## Key to Practice Figure

### Practice Figure 9.1

A. Crus cerebri, B. Locus coeruleus, C. Superior cerebellar peduncle, D. Middle cerebellar peduncle, E. Inferior cerebellar peduncle, F. Inferior fovea, G. Tuber cinereum, H. Cuneate tubercle, I. Gracile tubercle, J. Median sulcus, K. Superior fovea, L. Sulcus limitans, M. Facial colliculus, N. Vestibular area, O. Stria medullaris, P. Hypoglossal triangle, Q. Vagal triangle

## Key to MCQs

1. c 2. b 3. d 4. a 5. c 6. c 7. c
8. c 9. c 10. d 11. a

## Chapter 10

## Key to Clinicoanatomical Problem

### Clinical Case 1

1. a. Due to damage to the sensory relay nuclei within the thalamus.
   b. Due to abnormal processing of sensory information within the thalamocortical pathways which may lead to exaggerated responses to stimuli.
2. Thalamogeniculate branch of the posterior cerebral artery (PCA).

## Key to Practice Figures

### Practice Figure 10.1

A. Anterior nucleus, B. Intralaminar nuclei, C. External medullary lamina, D. Reticular nucleus, E. Ventral posteromedial nucleus (VPM), F. Interthalamic adhesion, G. Midline nuclei, H. Internal medullary lamina, I. Centromedian nucleus (CM), J. Medial geniculate body (MGB), K. Lateral geniculate body (LGB), L. Medial dorsal nucleus, M. Pulvinar

### Practice Figure 10.2

A. Septum pellucidum, B. Corpus callosum, C. Fornix containing choroid plexus, D. Anterior commissure, E. Third ventricle, F. Lamina terminalis, G. Optic recess, H. Infundibular recess, I. Mammillary body, J. Posterior perforated substance, K. Hypothalamic sulcus, L. Tela choroidea of third ventricle, M. Supraspinal recess, N. Great cerebral vein, O. Pineal body, P. Posterior commissure, Q. Fourth ventricle

## Key to MCQs

1. c 2. c 3. d 4. b 5. d 6. c 7. b
8. c 9. c 10. d 11. a 12. b 13. d 14. b
15. a 16. c

## Chapter 11

## Key to Clinicoanatomical Problem

### Clinical Case 1

1. Bradykinesia is difficulty in initiating and executing movements, leading to reduced spontaneous movements and overall motor activity.

2. Rigidity is an increase in muscle tone causing stiffness and resistance to movement.
3. Dopamine.

## Key to Practice Figures

### Practice Figure 11.1

A. Central sulcus, B. Postcentral gyrus, C. Postcentral sulcus, D. Intraparietal sulcus, E. Superior parietal lobule, F. Supramarginal gyrus, G. Angular gyrus, H. Parieto-occipital sulcus, I. Inferior parietal lobule, J. Lunate sulcus, K. Postcalcarine sulcus, L. Gyrus descendens, M. Inferior temporal sulcus, N. Middle temporal gyrus, O. Inferior temporal gyrus, P. Precentral gyrus, Q. Precentral sulcus, R. Superior frontal gyrus, S. Superior frontal sulcus, T. Middle frontal gyrus, U. Superior temporal gyrus, V. Inferior frontal sulcus, W. Pars opercularis of IFG, X. Anterior ascending ramus of LS, Y. Posterior ramus of LS, Z. Superior temporal sulcus

### Practice Figure 11.2

A. Fornix, B. Medial frontal gyrus, C. Cingulate sulcus, D. Cingulate gyrus, E. Callosal sulcus, F. Corpus callosum, G. Paraterminal gyrus, H. Posterior parolfactory sulcus, I. Parolfactory gyrus, J. Anterior parolfactory sulcus, K. Uncus, L. Rhinal sulcus, M. Parahippocampal gyrus, N. Paracentral lobule, O. Isthmus, P. Precuneus, Q. Suprasplenial sulcus, R. Parieto-occipital sulcus, S. Cuneus, T. Calcarine sulcus, U. Postcalcarine sulcus, V. Lingual gyrus, W. Collateral sulcus

### Practice Figure 11.3

A. Medial orbital gyrus, B. Olfactory sulcus, C. Gyrus rectus, D. Calcarine sulcus, E. Parieto-occipital sulcus, F. Cuneus, G. Anterior orbital gyrus, H. Lateral orbital gyrus, I. Posterior orbital gyrus, J. Rhinal sulcus, K. Uncus, L. Parahippocampal gyrus, M. Collateral sulcus, N. Medial occipitotemporal gyrus, O. Occipitotemporal sulcus, P. Lateral occipitotemporal gyrus, Q. Lingual gyrus, R. Lunate sulcus

### Practice Figure 11.4

A. Wernicke's sensory speech area, B. Visual areas (occipital lobe), C. Broca's motor speech area

### Practice Figure 11.5

A. Paracentral lobule, B. Ms 1, C. Ms 2, D. Cingulate gyrus, E. Uncus, F. Sm 1, G. Precuneus

### Practice Figure 11.6

A. Head of caudate nucleus, B. Anterior limb, C. Genu, D. Posterior limb, E. Thalamus, F. Tail of caudate nucleus, G. External capsule, H. Claustrum, I. Putamen, J. Globus Pallidus

### Practice Figure 11.7

A. Caudate nucleus (head), B. Anterior thalamic radiation (sensory), C. Corticonuclear fibres for head and neck (motor), D. Corticospinal fibres for upper limb (motor), E. Corticospinal fibres for trunk (motor), F. Corticospinal fibres for lower limb (motor), G. Superior thalamic radiation (sensory), H. Medial geniculate body, I. Lateral geniculate body, J. Frontopontine fibres (motor), K. Corticorubral fibres (motor), L. Auditory radiation (sensory)/inferior thalamic radiation, M. Parietopontine and occipitopontine fibres (motor), N. Optic radiation (sensory)/posterior thalamic radiation, O. Lentiform nucleus, P. Thalamus

## Key to MCQs

| | | | | | | |
|---|---|---|---|---|---|---|
| 1. a | 2. c | 3. b | 4. c | 5. d | 6. a | 7. c |
| 8. a | 9. b | 10. a | 11. c | 12. c | 13. a | 14. c |
| 15. b | 16. c | 17. d | | | | |

# Chapter 12

## Key to Clinicoanatomical Problem

### *Clinical Case 1*

1. Due to obstruction to normal flow of CSF out of the lateral ventricle through interventricular foramen. It leads to an accumulation of CSF in the lateral ventricles and subsequent dilation.
2. Due to increased intracranial pressure and CSF accumulation.

## Key to Practice Figures

### Practice Figure 12.1

A. Interventricular foramen, B. Anterior horn, C. Third ventricle, D. Inferior horn, E. Posterior horn, F. Fourth ventricle

### Practice Figure 12.2

A. Anterior horn of lateral ventricle, B. Corpus callosum, C. Head of caudate nucleus, D. Lentiform nucleus, E. Septum pellucidum, F. Column of fornix, G. Anterior commissure

### Practice Figure 12.3

A. Posterior horn of lateral ventricle, B. Bulb of the posterior horn, C. Forceps major, D. Tapetum, E. Optic radiation, F. Inferior longitudinal fasciculus, G. Calcar avis

### Practice Figure 12.4

A. Tail of caudate nucleus, B. Stria terminalis, C. Choroid plexus, D. Fimbria, E. Hippocampus, F. Collateral sulcus, G. Tapetum, H. Inferior horn of lateral ventricle, I. Collateral eminence, J. Temporal lobe

### Practice Figure 12.5

A. Columns of fornix, B. Mammillary bodies, C. Hippocampus, D. Body of fornix, E. Commissure of fornix, F. Crus of fornix, G. Dentate gyrus, H. Fimbria of hippocampus

## Key to MCQs

| | | | | | | |
|---|---|---|---|---|---|---|
| 1. a | 2. c | 3. b | 4. b | 5. d | 6. b | 7. c |
| 8. b | 9. c | 10. c | 11. c | 12. b | | |

# Chapter 13

## Key to MCQs

| | | | | | | |
|---|---|---|---|---|---|---|
| 1. b | 2. d | 3. d | 4. a | 5. d | 6. c | 7. b |
| 8. d | 9. d | 10. d | | | | |

# Chapter 14

## Key to Clinicoanatomical Problem

### *Clinical Case 1*

1. Because the lesion of internal capsule affected the corticospinal tract, responsible for motor control, and the corticobulbar tract, involved in speech and facial movements.
2. Lenticulostriate artery, a branch of the middle cerebral artery.

## Key to Practice Figures

### Practice Figure 14.1

A. Internal carotid artery, B. Anterior communicating artery, C. Recurrent artery of Heubner, D. Anterior cerebral artery, E. Ophthalmic artery, F. Middle cerebral artery, G. Anterior choroidal artery, H. Posterior communicating artery, I. Posterior cerebral artery, J. Posterior choroidal artery, K. Superior cerebellar artery, L. Basilar artery, M. Labyrinthine artery, N. Anterior inferior cerebellar artery, O. Vertebral artery, P. Anterior spinal artery, Q. Circle of Willis

### Practice Figure 14.2

A. Superior anastomotic vein (of Trolard), B. Inferior anastomotic vein (of Labbe), C. Transverse sinus, D. Sigmoid sinus, E. Superior cerebral veins, F. Superficial middle cerebral vein, G. Superior bulb of internal jugular vein, H. Internal jugular vein

## Key to MCQs

| | | | | | | |
|---|---|---|---|---|---|---|
| 1. c | 2. c | 3. b | 4. b | 5. d | 6. b | 7. d |
| 8. b | 9. c | 10. b | 11. d | 12. a | 13. c | 14. a |

# Chapter 15

## Key to Practice Figure

### Practice Figure 15.1

A. Frontal lobe, B. Lateral ventricle, C. Pineal gland (white dot), D. Occipital lobe

### Key to MCQs

1. a 2. b 3. c 4. d 5. b 6. d 7. a
8. c 9. b 10. a

## Chapter 16

### Key to Clinicoanatomical Problem

#### *Clinical Case 1*

1. Hirschsprung's disease.
2. Absence of ganglion cells in the colon.

### Key to MCQs

1. b 2. c 3. d 4. c 5. d 6. b 7. b
8. a 9. c 10. d

## Chapter 17

### Key to Clinicoanatomical Problem

#### *Clinical Case 1*

1. Spina bifida occulta has incompletely fused vertebral spine, but the spinal cord and its covering membranes typically remain in position.
2. Spina bifida is a neural tube defect that causes varying degrees of vertebral malformation.
3. Meningocele, myelomeningocele.

### Key to Practice Figure

#### Practice Figure 17.1

A. Skin, B. Meninges, C. Spinal cord, D. Tuft of hairs, E. Dimpling of skin, F. Meningeal sac, G. Spinal cord and spinal nerves in meningeal sac

### Key to MCQs

1. a 2. a 3. d 4. b 5. d 6. c 7. c
8. a 9. c 10. b 11. a 12. c 13. d

## Appendix

### Key to Spotters

#### *Spotter 1*

Stylohyoid, stylopharyngeus, styloglossus muscles, stylohyoid and stylomandibular ligaments.

#### *Spotter 2*

a. Typical cervical vertebra, b. Vertebral artery, the vertebral veins and a branch from the inferior cervical ganglion.

#### *Spotter 3*

a. Facial artery, b. Inferior labial, superior labial, lateral nasal branches.

#### *Spotter 4*

a. Mylohyoid muscle, b. Nerve to mylohyoid – branch of inferior alveolar branch of mandibular nerve.

#### *Spotter 5*

a. Sternocleidomastoid b. Spinal accessory nerve provides the motor supply, and branches from the ventral rami of C2 and C3 are proprioceptive.

#### *Spotter 6*

a. Hypoglossal nerve, b. Muscles of tongue except palatoglossus.

#### *Spotter 7*

a. Thyroid gland, b. Superior and inferior thyroid arteries, thyroidea ima artery.

#### *Spotter 8*

a. Oculomotor nerve, b. Superior rectus, inferior rectus, medial rectus and inferior oblique, levator palpebrae superioris.

#### *Spotter 9*

a. Epiglottis, b. Elastic cartilage.

#### *Spotter 10*

a. Hiatus semilunaris, b. Frontal, anterior ethmoidal and maxillary air sinuses.

#### *Spotter 11*

a. Thyroid cartilage, b. Hyaline cartilage.

#### *Spotter 12*

a. Circumvallate papillae, b. Glossopharyngeal nerve.

#### *Spotter 13*

a. Maxillary air sinus, b. in the posterior part of hiatus semilunaris, in the middle meatus of nose.

#### *Spotter 14*

a. Optic chiasma, b. Bitemporal hemianopia

#### *Spotter 15*

a. Corpus callosum, b. Rostrum, genu, body, splenium.

#### *Spotter 16*

a. Superior colliculus of midbrain, b. Oculomotor nucleus, Edinger-Westphal nucleus, mesencephalic nucleus of trigeminal nerve.

#### *Spotter 17*

a. Anterior horn of the lateral ventricle, b. Caudate nucleus.

#### *Spotter 18*

Facial colliculus, b. Motor nucleus of facial nerve and main sensory nucleus of trigeminal nerve

#### *Spotter 19*

a. Fourth ventricle, b. Hydrocephalus

#### *Spotter 20*

a. Precentral gyrus, b. Area 4

#### *Spotter 21*

a. Basilar artery, b. Pontine branches, anterior inferior cerebellar artery, labyrinthine artery, superior cerebellar artery, posterior cerebral artery.

#### *Spotter 22*

a. MRI, b. Corpus callosum.

#### *Spotter 23*

a. Carotis angiography, b. Internal carotid artery.

#### *Spotter 24*

a. Cerebellum, b. Vermis and cerebellar hemispheres.

#### *Spotter 25*

a. Filum terminale, b. Filum terminale internum and filum terminale externum.